Self-Assessment Colour Review

Wildlife Medicine & Rehabilitation

Anna L Meredith

MA, VetMB, CertLAS, DZooMed(Mammalian), MRCVS

and

Emma J Keeble

BVSc, DZooMed(Mammalian), MRCVS

RCVS Recognised Specialists in Zoo and Wildlife Medicine
Exotic Animal and Wildlife Service
Hospital for Small Animals
Royal (Dick) School of Veterinary Studies
University of Edinburgh
Easter Bush, Roslin, Scotland, UK

CRC Press
Taylor & Francis Group
6000 Broken Sound Parkway NW, Suite 300
Boca Raton, FL 33487-2742

© 2011 by Taylor & Francis Group, LLC
CRC Press is an imprint of Taylor & Francis Group, an Informa business

Visit the Taylor & Francis Web site at
http://www.taylorandfrancis.com

and the CRC Press Web site at
http://www.crcpress.com

Preface

Encounters with wildlife casualties are increasingly commonplace in veterinary practice. Whether these are due to natural disasters or man-made problems, there is a duty of care for the welfare of that animal. Initial assessment and triage are essential in the wildlife casualty case to enable decisions on treatment and rehabilitation methods to be made. These processes often involve a chain of veterinary personnel working closely with local or more specialized rehabilitators to facilitate the recuperation and eventual release back to the wild of the patient. Knowledge of the animal's unique biology, physiology and natural history is essential so that educated decisions can be made as to the best course of action. Difficult decisions may have to be made and these circumstances are covered in the text, with examples of cases where euthanasia may be indicated on welfare grounds.

The contributing authors have an enormous range of practical experience in their subject and this has resulted in a comprehensive and easy-to-use reference text. Common conditions seen in wildlife species in a range of different countries are covered, with cases from Europe, North America, the Middle East and Australia. It is obviously not possible to cover all species or conditions encountered, but we hope that the selection of cases presented covers sufficient common scenarios to have direct or indirect relevance to most readers. The book will appeal to veterinary professionals in general practice worldwide as a general reference text, and also for those working more directly with wildlife who wish to study this field in greater depth.

There are few textbooks available to the veterinary surgeon covering wildlife rehabilitation medicine in any detail. This book is designed to address that lack of information by providing the reader with an up-to-date text covering commonly presented conditions and species as well as providing more complex and unusual wildlife case material. It is not intended to be a comprehensive text and references are not provided.

We hope that readers will find this book both informative and enjoyable to read and that it will provide an easy revision text for testing existing knowledge and be of help to those revising for postgraduate examinations.

Anna Meredith
Emma Keeble

Acknowledgements

The editors are very grateful for the expertise, hard work and punctuality of all the authors. We would also like to thank Jill Northcott, Michael Manson and the team at Manson Publishing for all their encouragement, patience and technical assistance. In particular we would like to thank our partners and families for all their support and encouragement over the past year.

Picture acknowledgements

8 courtesy of British Divers Marine Life Rescue

18, 30, 174, 186, 192a, 194a, 198 and 202 courtesy of Secret World Wildlife Rescue

21 courtesy of Mary-Anne Barnett

33a courtesy of Declan O'Donovan

43, 68, 133, 177a and 177b courtesy of Kevin Eatwell

62 courtesy of Institute of Zoology

67a, 67b, 67c, 95a and 95b courtesy of Scott Fitzgerald

75c courtesy of Sherry Morgan

76 courtesy of Jim Sikarskie

78a, 78b and 78c courtesy of Michael Pyne

81b courtesy of Joerg Kinne

91b courtesy of Lorraine Fleming

101b courtesy of Christudas Silvanose

115b courtesy of Central Veterinary Research Laboratory, Dubai

142 reprinted with permission from Samour JH (2000) (ed) *Avian Medicine*. Mosby, London, pp.181–186

148b reprinted with permission from *Journal of Zoo and Wildlife Medicine* (1997) 28:325–330

155a and 155b courtesy of Frank Slansky

183 courtesy of Roger Musgrove

Contributors

Tom A Bailey BVSc, BSc, PhD, MSc, CertZooMed, MRCVS
Dubai Falcon Hospital, Dubai, United Arab Emirates

James E F Barnett BVSc, BSc, MRCVS
British Divers Marine Life Rescue, Uckfield, East Sussex, UK

J R Best BVMS, MRCVS
Ashford, Kent, UK

Steve Bexton BVMS, CertZooMed, MRCVS
RSPCA Norfolk Wildlife Hospital, East Winch, Kings Lynn Norfolk, UK

Suzetta Billington BSc, BVSc, MSc, MRCVS
Birch Heath Veterinary Clinic, Tarporley, Cheshire, UK

Debra C Bourne MA, VetMB, PhD, MRCVS
Beckenham, Kent, UK

Michelle L Campbell-Ward BVSc, BSc, DZooMed (Mammalian), MRCVS
Taronga Conservation Society Australia, Dubbo, New South Wales, Australia

John R Chitty BVetMed, CertZooMed, MRCVS
JC Exotic Pet Consultancy, Salisbury, Wiltshire, UK

Glen O Cousquer BVM&S, BSc(Hons), CertZooMed, PGDOE, MSc, MRCVS
Moray House School of Education, University of Edinburgh, Edinburgh, UK

Simon R Hollamby BVSc, DiplACZM, MRCVS
Toronto Zoo, Toronto, Ontario, Canada

Emma J Keeble BVSc, DZooMed(Mammalian), MRCVS
Easter Bush Veterinary Centre, University of Edinburgh, Roslin, UK

Becki Lawson BA, VetMB, MRCVS
Brixton, London, UK

Lesa A Longley BVM&S, DZooMed(Mammalian), MRCVS
Penicuik, Midlothian, UK

Erica Miller DVM
Tri-State Bird Rescue and Research, Inc., Newark, Delaware, USA

Elizabeth Mullineaux BVM&S, CertSHP, MRCVS
Quantock Veterinary Hospital, Bridgewater, Somerset, UK

Maria L Parga DVM, MSc
SUBMON, Barcelona, Spain

Ian Robinson BVSc, CertSHP, CertZooMed, FRCVS
International Fund for Animal Welfare, Yarmouth Port, Massachusetts, USA

Andrew D Routh BVSc, CertZooMed, MRCVS
Zoological Society of London, Regent's Park, London, UK

Richard A Saunders BVSc, BSc, DZooMed (Mammalian), MRCVS
Veterinary Department, Bristol Zoo Gardens, Bristol, UK

Colin Seddon
SSPCA, Middlebank Wildlife Centre, Dunfermline, Fife, UK

Victor R Simpson BVSc, DTVM, CBiol, FIBiol, FRCVS
Truro, Cornwall, UK

Jonathan M Sleeman MA, VetMB, DipACZM, MRCVS
USGS National Wildlife Health Center, Madison, Wisconsin, USA

Alexandra J Tomlinson MA, VetMB, MRCVS
Wildlife and Emerging Diseases Programme, FERA, Stonehouse, Gloucestershire, UK

Katherine E Whitwell BVSc, DipECVP, FRCVS
Equine Pathology Consultancy, Newmarket, Suffolk, UK

Classification of cases

Flamingos
1, 65

Swans, ducks, geese
4, 7, 25, 29, 51, 80, 90, 117, 118, 133,
140, 145, 151, 157, 166, 175, 179, 182,
192

Buzzards, kestrels, sparrowhawks,
falcons, vultures, eagles
5, 23, 37, 42, 59, 81, 88, 109, 116, 121,
137, 147, 156, 160, 162, 188

Owls
10, 41, 53, 79, 96, 123, 153, 168, 199,
201, 204

Blackbirds, greenfinches, chaffinches
24, 31, 48, 63, 169, 177, 184

Ospreys
26, 77

Guillemots, curlews, gulls
27, 46, 134, 181

Pheasants
35

Lorikeets
78

Herons
98

Bustards, coots, moorhens
101, 102, 115, 127, 135, 142, 148, 152

Cuckoos
170

Doves
190, 197

Squirrels
2, 36, 75, 126, 155, 159

Hares, rabbits
6, 18, 22, 39, 55, 68, 100, 110, 122,
132, 161, 189

Foxes, otters, badgers, raccoons, mink
11, 14, 17, 30, 38, 45, 49, 54, 60, 69,
85, 103, 106, 107, 119, 131, 138, 146,
163, 172, 176, 180, 191, 193, 194, 198

Hedgehogs
12, 13, 32, 57, 64, 86, 87, 125, 136,
158, 165, 185, 196, 205

Seals
3, 16, 19, 61, 70, 72, 73, 91, 94, 128,
129, 143, 178

Dolphins, whales
8, 9, 21, 28, 62, 104

Manatees
15

Hippopotami, oryx, deer
20, 33, 34, 43, 59, 67, 71, 93, 95, 99,
108, 124, 150, 164, 174, 202

Gorillas
50, 130

Elephants
76

Bats
89, 112, 141, 182

Shrew
97

Echidna
120

Wallabies, possums, kangaroos, koalas
44, 92, 171, 195, 206

Reptiles
40, 52, 74, 83, 105, 144, 149

Miscellaneous
47, 56, 66, 82, 84, 111, 113, 114, 139,
154, 167, 173, 186, 187, 200, 203

1 A four-month-old greater flamingo presented with a lesion involving the dorsal eyelid (1). The bird was housed outside in a park with a group of 20 other chicks of similar age. A further four chicks had similar lesions on the non-feathered skin of their hock joints or on the feathered part of their necks.

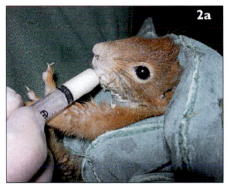

i. List the differential diagnoses for these lesions.
ii. What are the diagnostic test(s) to determine a provisional diagnosis and to confirm the diagnosis?
iii. What therapeutic and surgical considerations are there, and what is the prognosis in this case?
iv. What preventive measures can be taken to avoid this condition?

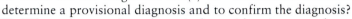

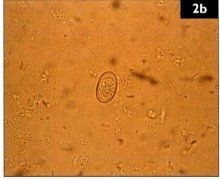

2 An orphaned juvenile red squirrel develops pale yellow diarrhoea while being hand-reared (2a). Direct microscopy (×100) of a faecal smear reveals a few small oval structures (2b).
i. What is the organism shown?
ii. Is this likely to be causing the diarrhoea?
iii. What factors could be contributing to the diarrhoea and how could these be reduced?

1 i. Mosquito bites, mite infestations, haematomas, early abscesses, avipox infection, mycobacteriosis, neoplasia. This was a case of cutaneous avipox.

ii. A provisional diagnosis can be made based of clinical signs. A definitive diagnosis is made histopathologically, with examination of biopsy samples and demonstration of typical intracytoplasmic inclusions or Bollinger bodies. Virus isolation using biopsy samples is possible using the chorioallantoic membrane of embryonated chicken eggs. Electron microscopy is important because it is not always possible to isolate virus from dry scabs.

iii. There is no specific treatment. Secondary infection with bacteria or fungi may be treated with broad-spectrum antibacterial or antifungal therapy. Supplementation with vitamin A to promote epithelial regeneration and topical antibacterial/antifungal creams or mercurochrome may be helpful. Hydrocolloid or hydroactive dressings will aid skin healing. Electrocautery and chemical cautery using silver nitrate pencils can be used to treat cutaneous lesions. Large proliferative lesions may need to be surgically excised. In mild cases the prognosis is good. Large pox lesions involving the eyelids or diphtheritic oropharyngeal lesions interfere with vision and feeding and leave permanent scars. Scabs around a digit can lead to constriction injuries and loss of digits. Scabs on eyelids can cause keratitis and corneal ulceration.

iv. There are no commercially available flamingo pox vaccines. Mosquito control should include netting around the area where the birds are housed. Clinical cases should be isolated.

2 i. A coccidial oocyst (*Eimeria* spp.)

ii. Coccidia are commonly found in the intestine of red squirrels and are usually non-pathogenic; however, they can cause disease in stressed or immunosuppressed animals.

iii. Poor husbandry and management in captivity could be contributing to the diarrhoea. Red squirrels are nervous animals prone to stress in captivity, especially if being regularly handled. Stress should be reduced by keeping human contact to a minimum and keeping the squirrel in a warm quiet secluded environment. A nest box should be provided to make it feel more secure. Ideally, only one person should be responsible for feeding the squirrel and it should be handled confidently and gently. If kept with or near other squirrels, then competition, dominance or aggression might be causing stress. Strict hygiene is essential, especially in the areas where food is available. The milk replacer and any supplementary food should be fresh and suitable for red squirrels, and any changes to the diet gradually introduced.

3 A harbour seal was admitted into rehabilitation as an abandoned dependent pup. Rehabilitation proceeded uneventfully for about three weeks, during which time the seal was fed on a liquid diet by gavage tube. The seal then started the weaning process, involving the introduction of assist-fed whole fish. Immediately on the introduction of whole fish, the seal showed intermittent

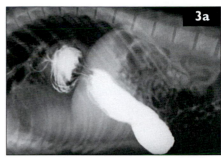

distress on assisted feeding. Some fish were regurgitated immediately after feeding, others vomited within 30 minutes. Occasionally, feeding would progress without incident or vomiting.

Clinical examination revealed no abnormality and the animal was within normal weight range for the stage of rehabilitation. All standard blood parameters were normal. Plain radiographs of the chest and abdomen were unremarkable. 150 ml of barium contrast medium was delivered into the caudal oesophagus via gavage tube and a radiograph (3a) taken within five minutes.

i. What can you see on the radiograph?
ii. What is your diagnosis?
iii. When considering possible treatment options, what must be taken into consideration?
iv. Why are plain radiographs in seals often unrevealing?

4 You are presented with a young adult mute swan found this morning by the side of a road. The weather is wet and windy. On examination the swan has a slightly wide-based gait, is moderately underweight and has scuffed plantar feet and hocks, a wound on the skin over the keel bone and some bruising to the upper bill. The appearance of the wound, several days after débriding, is shown (4).

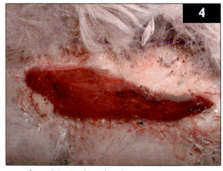

i. What are the possible differential diagnoses for this individual?
ii. What diagnostic tests might you perform?
iii. How would you treat such a wound in this species?

3 i. A diaphragmatic hernia of the cardiac area of the stomach. A dilated caudal oesophagus, lightly outlined by barium and filled with air, is also visible. ii. Diaphragmatic hernia and megaloesophagus (confirmed on necropsy, 3b). iii. The diaphragmatic hernia might be operable and the megaloesophagus may respond to conservative treatment,

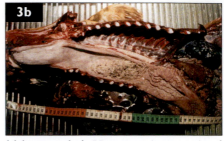

although the prognosis for recovery would be guarded. However, in an animal intended for return to the wild, there are three major considerations:
- Possible interference with the diaphragmatic sphincter, which controls the flow of deoxygenated blood from the hepatic vein back to the heart during prolonged breath holding (part of the 'dive reflex') by surgical correction of the hernia could have severe repercussions for the seal;
- Significant risk of breakdown of a surgical repair during deep diving due to increased pressure on organs;
- This is a congenital and possibly hereditary condition. Should the seal survive and breed, it could propagate the condition in the wild population.

iv. Because of the lack of intra-abdominal fat. Although the percentage of fat to body mass in seals is similar to land mammals, the fat is concentrated in the blubber layer for insulation.

4 i. This has been caused either by a single traumatic event or because of a period of time spent in ventral recumbency on hard surfacing. The history is strongly suggestive of impact trauma (swans may land on wet roads, mistaking them for water) given the typical foot lesions.

ii. Swans suffering from lead poisoning are more likely to fly into power cables and other objects. It would therefore be advisable to screen for lead poisoning by gizzard radiography and blood lead analysis. Survey radiographs, especially of the pelvis, would be advised given the gait abnormality.

iii. The wound appears relatively superficial and to be healing well after débridement. Protective dressings, adherent to the skin or sutured into place, encourage granulation and offer physical protection while helping to keep the wound clean. More chronic or deeper wounds are challenging to treat. They may require repeated débridement, possibly even including bone. Avian skin is thin and inelastic; this area continues to be traumatized by contact with substrate, and the keel bone itself applies further localized pressure to the healing area. Thick bedding, protective dressings, systemic antibiosis and analgesia are all helpful. Swans rarely self-mutilate. The prognosis is guarded.

5 This buzzard (**5a**) was brought in to the veterinary clinic by a member of the public. It was lethargic and anorexic and died shortly after examination.
i. Describe the lesions shown.
ii. What is the cause of this problem, and what treatment should be instituted?

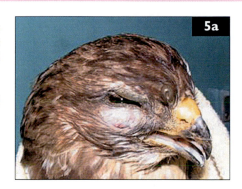

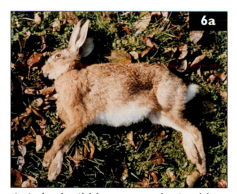
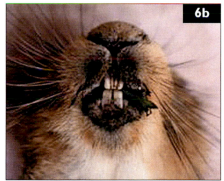

6 A dead wild hare was submitted by a gamekeeper (**6a**). It was in an emaciated, dehydrated state with no evidence of diarrhoea. Fur around the mouth was darkened and matted and green food protruded, but there was no lip ulceration (**6b**). Palpation of the abdomen revealed very firm abdominal contents that subsequently proved to be due to the dehydration of the large bowel contents, which moulded to the folds in the wall. In addition, the stomach was distended and there were minimal internal body fat reserves. The lower lobes of the lungs were congested and firm due to inhalation pneumonia.
i. What condition is suggested by these external features?
ii. How would you investigate it further?
iii. Is this a common condition?
iv. Has it been seen in rabbits?
v. What is the cause of the condition?

5 i. There is severe localized soft tissue swelling associated with oedema and subcutaneous haemorrhage surrounding the right eye.

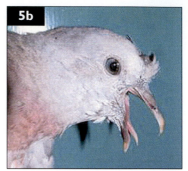

ii. A large engorged *Ixodid* tick. There is an association between tissue oedema/haemorrhage and the presence of engorged adult female ticks. *Ixodes frontalis* is a specific avian parasite that has been reported in France and the UK, although concurrent infection with *Borrelia burgdorferi* has also been implicated. Its preferred habitat is bushes, brambles and hedges, and bird species frequenting these habitats may be more likely to develop tick-related syndrome (TRS). Raptors, Turdidae and Columbiformes (e.g. the collared dove shown in 5b) appear to be more commonly affected. TRS is poorly understood. Acute death, lethargy, depression, focal swelling and/or haemorrhage are all typically seen. It has been suggested that free-living species may be more resistant to TRS, either innately or due to previous exposure. TRS may also render individuals more vulnerable to other problems that mask signs of TRS.

The use of broad-spectrum antibiotics, together with anti-inflammatories, is recommended. Supportive fluid and nutritional therapy should be provided as part of the treatment plan. Any engorged ticks should be removed and an ectoparasiticide, such as fipronil, used for the treatment and prevention of tick infestations.

6 i. Leporine dysautonomia. Perioral matting of fur occurs in 58% of cases due to defective swallowing, gastric distension in 65% and large bowel impaction in 97% of cases. At the time of death, 87% show atrophy of body fat reserves and 52% have developed inhalation pneumonia.
ii. Histological examination of ganglionic neurons (left cranial mesenteric and the stellate ganglia are the easiest to locate). In positive cases, some chromatolytic degenerate neurons are present within the ganglia.
iii. Dysautonomia was the second commonest cause of death in one survey, causing 24% of the hare deaths.
iv. Yes. Dysautonomia has been confirmed in two young wild rabbits and in some cases of constipative mucoid enteropathy in domestic rabbits.
v. Unknown. The condition shares features with equine grass sickness. The current belief is that equine dysautonomia may be associated with a form of botulism.

7 A juvenile mute swan of abnormal appearance has been noticed with an apparent deformity of the wings (7).
i. What is this condition commonly called?
ii. What has caused this abnormality?
iii. How will this affect the swan in the wild?
iv. What can be done to treat this condition?

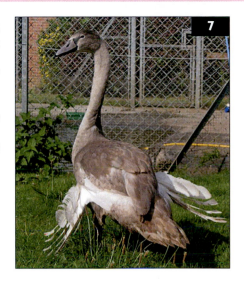

8 A cetacean (the Atlantic white-sided dolphin shown in 8) strands on a beach and you are the veterinary surgeon called to the scene. What are the possible reasons for this animal stranding?

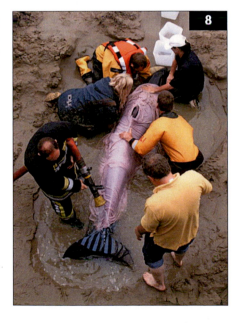

7 **i.** Angel wing; also slipped wing, flip wing and straw wing.
ii. An angular limb deformity, which occurs during the period of rapid flight feather growth if the bones of the carpus are not strong enough. The increasing weight of the developing feathers causes carpal valgus and lateral rotation, resulting in the primary feathers being inverted and laterally protruding when the wing is folded. Although genetic factors may be involved, the primary mechanism is excessive dietary protein during the period of primary feather growth, leading to increasing feather weight before the appendicular skeleton is sufficiently ossified to support it.
iii. Affected birds are permanently flightless and, therefore, less able to escape from territorial attack by other swans and at increased risk from predation. The primary feathers often become traumatized and frayed at the ends due to the angle at which they stick out. Despite this, birds in suitable environments can thrive well.
iv. If noticed early enough, while the bones are still growing, some mild deformities will respond to corrective bandaging and splints. Once the bones are ossified, the changes are irreversible without surgical osteotomy and intramedullary pinning of the metacarpal bone. This usually restores the cosmetic appearance of the wing, but will not necessarily restore full flight status.

8 Pelagic and coastal species of cetacean may live strand due to disease, leaving them weak and disorientated. Infectious disease conditions commonly reported include lungworm and/or bacterial pneumonia, bacterial septicaemia and meningoencephalitis. Non-infectious conditions encountered include starvation/hypothermia and trauma. A certain number of primarily pelagic dolphins and whales also appear to strand in relatively healthy condition with no evidence of significant pathology (coastal species such as harbour porpoises rarely do so). Theories for this are focussed on navigational error. Distortion of echolocation signals, the system of sonar used by beaked whales and dolphins to catch prey and navigate, may occur in shallow water, particularly on gently shelving beaches. Pelagic dolphins also may be stranded by the receding tide when chasing prey inshore. Some scientists believe cetaceans use geomagnetic contours to navigate, with increased frequency of strandings where these contours cross the coast perpendicularly. Links also have been made between the mass stranding of beaked whales and the use of military active sonar. Mass strandings are thought to occur as a consequence of strong social ties in gregarious species (e.g. long-finned pilot whales and Atlantic white-sided dolphins), leading to the stranding of entire social groups after one individual strands for any of the reasons outlined above.

9 What are the options available for management of the stranded cetacean shown in **8**?

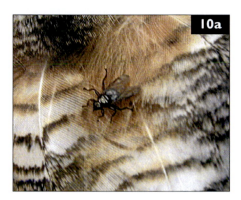

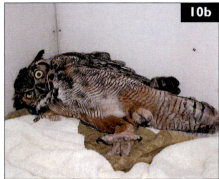

10 An immature great horned owl is found in late August by the side of the road. Physical examination reveals no external injuries, thin body condition (weight 760 g), several hippoboscid flies (**10a**), moderate dehydration, intermittent torticollis and mild ataxia when placed in a cage. Radiographs and a fundic examination are within normal limits. Stabilization care consists of

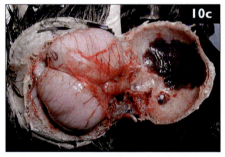

intravenous lactated Ringer's solution, systemic NSAIDs and oral rehydrating solution. The bird becomes profoundly neurological over the next several hours (sternal recumbency, rolling and eventually seizuring) (**10b**), produces watery, foul diarrhoea and dies. Necropsy reveals a thin bird with little to no fat reserves, no food in the upper GI tract and otherwise grossly normal tissues with the exception of the brain (**10c**).

i. What conditions would be on the initial list of differentials?
ii. What is the significance of the gross lesions in the brain?
iii. Is there a zoonotic concern with this case or any concern for other birds in-house?

9 Refloatation, rehabilitation and euthanasia. With prompt action and careful assessment, refloatation is appropriate for some pelagic animals that live strand, specifically those that strand in relatively healthy condition. Refloatation is used widely in New Zealand, which has a large number of live strandings annually and where the majority strand in a healthy state. In a number of other countries, cetacean experts argue against the use of refloatation as an option for the management of particularly single stranded cetaceans, as clinical assessment on the beach is not ideal and response may not always be immediate. Onset of shock, organ failure and muscle damage following stranding are insidious and these life-threatening sequelae occur regardless of condition at the time of stranding and worsen the longer the animal remains out of the water.

Rehabilitation requires facilities that include: an oval or round pool over 2 m deep and 9 m in diameter (to allow free swimming during recovery), with an adequately filtered/treated and temperature-controlled salt water supply; isolation from other marine mammals; facilities available for handling, feeding and treatment. In Europe, facilities are found in the Netherlands and Spain, and there are several in the USA. Survival rates vary considerably between facilities. There are limits on the size of animal that can be taken into rehabilitation.

10 i. Head trauma (hit by vehicle), cholinesterase inhibition (organophosphate or carbamate toxicity), heavy metal toxicity, West Nile virus (WNV) infection, bacterial or fungal meningitis, cerebral nematodiasis and toxoplasmosis, among others. The chronicity (thin bird), lack of external injuries, diarrhoea and presence of hippoboscid flies are strongly suggestive of WNV infection.
ii. Gross haemorrhage in the brain is commonly, though not consistently, seen with WNV encephalitis in birds. It is often misinterpreted as gross evidence of head trauma.
iii. WNV in birds can be transmitted to humans, though the incidence is quite low (transmission has occurred through scalpel injuries during necropsies and possibly through exposure of body fluids to human mucous membranes). Transmission to other birds, via fecal ingestion or via vectors (mosquitoes and hippoboscid flies), is a greater concern. Precautions, including parasite control, isolation of suspected cases and good personal hygiene, should be taken to minimize this possible transmission.

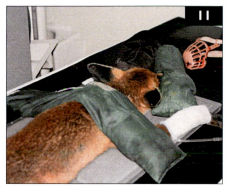

11 You are presented with an unconscious fox (**11**) that has recently been involved in a road traffic accident (RTA).
i. What would be your immediate care of this case?
ii. The following day the fox is conscious. How would you continue your assessment of it?

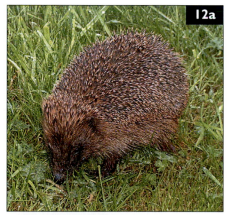

12 A hedgehog is discovered by a client it in his garden during the daytime. It is mild weather in late October in central England. The hedgehog (**12a**) weighs approximately 350 g, and has a rasping cough.
i. What is the most likely aetiology for this condition?
ii. How would you diagnose and treat it?

11 i. As the fox is unconscious, it is may be possible to make a full clinical examination, but this should not compromise human safety. Using a Baskerville-type dog muzzle will prevent unexpected bites. The species (red fox), age (adult) and sex (male) of the fox should be noted. An assessment of the body condition (good) should be made and the fox examined for evidence of chronic disease. Further diagnostic tests may be indicated. Immediate basic first aid treatment might include fluid therapy, analgesia, broad-spectrum antibiotics, provision of warmth and oxygen. The fox should be hospitalized and monitored in a quiet environment away from the sounds of people and other animals.

ii. When the fox is conscious it will be more difficult to handle, but easier to assess. Because of the previous loss of consciousness, a full assessment of locomotion and mental status are necessary. Remote cameras are a useful aid. If clinical problems are evident, examination under sedation or anaesthesia may be necessary once the animal is clinically stable. A suitable rehabilitation facility is likely to be required for several days. Once considered fit for release, RTA casualties should be returned to the site at which they were found.

12 i. Lungworm infestation (with the species *Crenosoma striatum* and/or *Capillaria aerophila*). The typical bipolar *Capillaria* egg in a faeces sample is shown (**12b**). *Crenosoma* are typically seen as first-stage larvae and may be seen live or dead in the faeces after being coughed up and swallowed. Intestinal capillariasis is also possible.

ii. Examine a faeces sample microscopically as a fresh wet preparation. A negative sample does not disprove the possibility of infestation, due to the intermittent shedding of eggs and larvae. A sputum sample may be obtained, under general anaesthesia, via swab or endotracheal tube from the trachea. A number of commonly used anthelminthics are effective against these species. The most effective regime appears to be levamisole (27 mg/kg s/c on alternate days for 3 doses). Concurrent bacterial bronchopneumonia is common, and inflammation and the presence of exudate and dead or dying worms can worsen the animal's respiratory condition. Broad-spectrum antibiotics and bromhexine, clenbuterol, etamiphylline and dembrexin can be used both systemically and by nebulization; however, titration of drugs designed for large animals is potentially very inaccurate. Glucocorticoids or NSAIDs may be of benefit to reduce the hypersensitivity reactions associated with lungworm die-off and reduce inflammation.

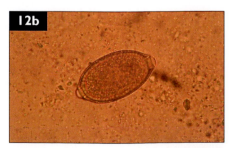
12b

13 What ancillary treatment might you provide for the hedgehog in 12, and how would you advise caring for this animal and releasing it?

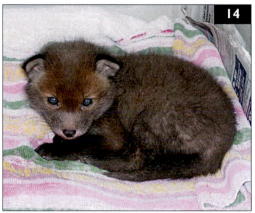

14 A small fox cub is discovered above ground at dusk with no vixen in sight. It is taken into captivity (14).
i. What is the likelihood of it having been abandoned?
ii. What two natural situations could explain the appearance of apparently abandoned fox cubs above ground?
iii. What are the main long-term behavioural problems that may be caused by hand-rearing fox cubs?
iv. What is the most common congenital abnormality of fox cubs, which often results in maternal rejection?
v. What should be done with this fox cub?

13 Hedgehogs are simple to care for in captivity in the short term and can be fed on a mixture of dried and tinned dog and cat foods, although proprietary hedgehog foods exist. The addition to, or replacement of, such a diet with live invertebrate prey, insectivorous bird foods and chopped day-old chicks provides a more naturalistic diet. Younger hedgehogs may benefit from the addition of pancreatic enzyme preparations to increase the digestibility of proprietary diets. Release should be delayed until the animal weighs at least 500 g, during a spell of warm weather or the end of the winter. If necessary, the hedgehog should be overwintered until the spring. Release should ideally be associated with provision of some supplementary food for a few days, in a suitable environment, lacking predators, far from roads and with nesting areas.

14 i. Fox cubs are very rarely abandoned and will usually have their mother nearby. Genuinely orphaned cubs are usually thin, weak and vocal.
ii. Weaned cubs are often seen above ground playing and learning survival skills without the obvious presence of the vixen. Litters of younger cubs less than four weeks old are sometimes translocated by the vixen to safer sites, and one or two may be left behind while she moves the others. The vixen will usually return later.
iii. It is difficult to rear fox cubs in captivity and ensure that they acquire the necessary hunting and social skills to survive back in the wild afterwards. The species is prone to becoming tame and imprinted on humans, so it is imperative to keep all human contact to a minimum, keep cubs in small groups of similar ages, and feed natural food (e.g carrion from road kill) to develop natural dietary tastes. At about six weeks old, cubs should be kept in a large enclosure with environmental enrichment to encourage the development of natural behaviour.
iv. Hydrocephalus.
v. The cub should be handled as little as possible and, if healthy, returned to where it was found, if safe from people and dogs. The area should be checked the following day to ensure that it has been retrieved by the vixen.

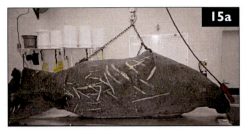

15 The dorsal surface of a Florida manatee demonstrating propeller wounds is shown (15a). Briefly describe the common reasons for presentation of manatees in their habitat off the coastal waters of Florida, USA, to specialist manatee rehabilitation centres.

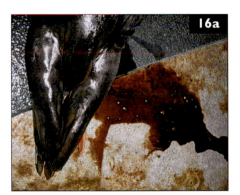 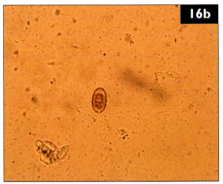

16 A group of juvenile common seals in a rehabilitation centre suddenly develop greenish-brown watery diarrhoea (16a) and become dull, lethargic and inappetent. Examination of faeces by direct microscopy reveals large numbers of organisms (16b), approximately 45 × 25 μm.
i. What are these organisms?
ii. How significant are they?
iii. What management factors could have contributed to their presence?
iv. What are the other principal differential diagnoses for diarrhoea in these seals?

15 Boat collision injuries are one of the most common reasons for presentation to rehabilitation facilities. Propeller blade injuries can penetrate the pleural cavity, with secondary bacterial infections and sepsis often proving fatal. Internally, the manatee's body cavity is divided longitudinally, with each dorsally located lung further separated by hemidiaphragms. Fistulous tracts and chronic vertebral osteomyelitis are com-

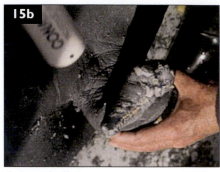

mon sequelae. Blunt trauma associated with boat hull impact can cause pneumothorax, pyothorax, pulmonary haemorrhage and secondary buoyancy problems. Traumatic injuries are also caused by entanglement with fishing lines, crab pots and other discarded debris and waste. When severe, these injuries may cause, or require, pectoral flipper amputation (15b). Orphaned or abandoned neonatal manatees usually present cachexic, dehydrated and hypoglycaemic, with major metabolic abnormalities. Sepsis and secondary skin infections are common. Juvenile manatees (<300 kg) and adults are prone to cold stress in cooler waters (<20°C) and present similarly to orphaned neonates. Outbreaks of *Karenia brevis*, commonly known as red tide, have caused mass mortality events in manatees. This dinoflagellate produces a potent neurotoxin termed brevetoxin. Clinical signs noted include dyspnoea, flaccid paralysis, muscle fasciculations, hyperflexion, disorientation and seizures. Chronic abscessation of the dermis and deeper muscle planes is a common problem in rehabilitating manatees.

16 i. *Eimeria phocae* oocysts.
ii. Occasionally, small numbers of oocysts are found in seal faeces with little significance; however, the large numbers found in these seals are likely to be causing enterocolitis, resulting in diarrhoea and occasionally dysentery.
iii. A build-up of sporulated oocysts in the environment is more likely in conditions of overcrowding and poor hygiene. Increased temperature and humidity also favour the survival of oocysts.
iv. Sudden diet change, especially a change to poorer quality fish; stress (e.g. recent changes to their captive environment); bacterial enteritis (e.g. *Clostridium perfringens*, salmonellosis, coliform enteritis); severe gastrointestinal helminthiasis; viral enteritis.

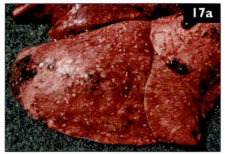

17 You carry out a post-mortem examination on an otter killed in a road traffic accident and observe that there are numerous whitish lesions about 1 mm in diameter scattered throughout the lungs (17a).
i. What would be your provisional diagnosis?
ii. How would you try to confirm this?
iii. What is the clinical significance of the disease?

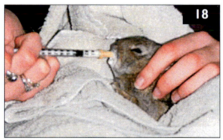

18 You are presented with a litter of orphaned wild rabbits approximately 10 days old (18).
i. How would you initially feed these animals?
ii. At what age would you introduce weaning food, and what would you consider to be suitable food items?
iii. What problems may be associated with hand-rearing rabbits, and how might these be overcome?

17 i. Adiaspiromycosis, a condition caused by the dimorphic fungus *Emmonsia crescens*. In its free-living or saprophytic state the fungus grows on decaying plant material, where it produces numerous small spores, 2–4 µm diameter, called conidiospores. If these are inhaled, they develop in the lung parenchyma and form thick-walled spores known as adiaspores. Adiaspores

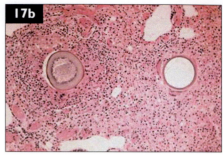

can grow up to 500 µm in diameter, but do not divide or develop further in the mammalian host. They are released back into the environment only when the host dies or is eaten by a predator. The adiaspores become surrounded by inflammatory cells and it is these that form the characteristic lesion. A major differential diagnosis is tuberculosis.

ii. Histopathological examination. Adiaspores surrounded by granulomatous reaction in an otter's lung are shown in this H&E-stained section (**17b**).

iii. Adiaspiromycosis is a common condition of animals that hunt or nest underground. It is rarely of clinical significance, but the lesions can closely resemble those of tuberculosis. Although humans can become infected, this is only by inhalation of spores from the environment. Adiaspiromycosis is not a zoonosis.

18 i. In the wild, suckling lagomorphs take large feeds, usually just once a day. Hand-reared rabbits should be fed 3–6 times a day on a suitable replacement milk feed, such as commercial dog and cat milk replacers or goats milk. Volumes of feed will depend on age and frequency of feeding.

ii. Wild rabbits begin to wean at 2–3 weeks old. An assortment of grass, fresh leaves and leafy vegetables should be provided together with ad-libitum hay. A commercial 'junior' pelleted food can also be used.

iii. Problems include aspiration pneumonia, digestive disturbances and diarrhoea during the milk feeding phase. These can be prevented by good hygiene, as well as a careful feeding technique. Coccidiosis may be a problem in groups of young rabbits. At weaning, fatal digestive disturbances and diarrhoea are common and these are attributed to a lack of access to adult caecotrophs, which establish normal gut flora. Feeding of fresh caecotrophs from healthy adults and the use of probiotics have been advocated.

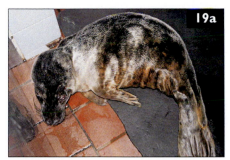

19 This juvenile grey seal pup is brought to a wildlife hospital for veterinary assessment. On examination it is found to be emaciated (based on visibly distinct neck, pelvis and ribs and evidence of loose skin) and dehydrated (19a).
i. How may dehydration be assessed on clinical examination in this species?
ii. What is the recommended route for fluid therapy in this animal, and what site is most commonly used?

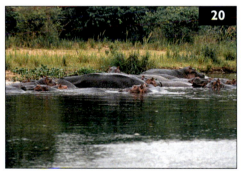

20 In 2004/2005 an outbreak of anthrax (*Bacillus anthracis*) killed 306 hippopotami in the Queen Elizabeth National Park in western Uganda (20). This mortality represented 11.63% of the total park hippo population.
i. Give a list of possible differential diagnoses for sudden death in this group of hippos.
ii. Describe possible modes of transmission that would sustain this anthrax outbreak.
iii. What management actions would you recommend to respond to this outbreak, and how would you dispose of affected carcasses?

19 i. Dehydrated seal pups have sunken eyes and dry mucous membranes and lack normal tear staining around the eyes. The 'skin pinch test' is unreliable due to the tight application of the skin to the blubber layer. Normal hydrated pups have wetness around the eyes due to tear staining, since nasolacrimal ducts are absent.

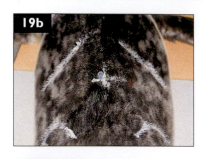

ii. The extradural intravertebral vein is located with the seal pup restrained in sternal recumbency. Access to this vein is best achieved midline via the L3/L4 intervertebral space at a distance halfway between the caudal most ribs and the iliac crests (**19b**). In pups weighing <25 kg the anatomical landmarks can be palpated to aid location of the site. A 21 gauge 2.5–5 cm needle is inserted perpendicular to the skin and advanced until blood appears in the hub. Correct placement can be confirmed by

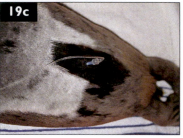

drawing blood back first. The needle is left *in situ* and an intravenous fluid giving set is attached (**19c**). Once the animal is hydrated it will start to move around more and alternative fluid therapy routes will need to be employed.

20 i. Botulism, toxicities (both natural and anthropogenic), anthrax, peracute babesiosis and theileriosis (East Coast fever).

ii. (1) Contamination of hippo grazing tracks with blood from infected animals. Hippos tend to use well worn tracks for their nocturnal terrestrial grazing habits. (2) Ingestion of spore-contaminated stagnant water in small pools. (3) Spore contamination of open wounds. Hippos are very aggressive and aquatically territorial with fight wounds being common. (4) Ingestion of infected carcasses. Cannibalism has been reported to occur in hippos. (5) Mechanical transmission through biting haematophagous flies

iii. Anthrax may be seen as part of the natural ecology of endemic areas. However, intervention may be required due to its zoonotic implications (at least 4–7 people are reported to have died in this outbreak after eating contaminated hippo meat), its effects on domestic livestock (many livestock graze on the periphery or within national parks in East Africa) and its effects on endangered species of wildlife. Management actions used in this outbreak were carcass disposal by cremation or burying under a layer of quicklime, vaccination of at-risk local livestock and education of local communities. Anthrax is a notifiable disease in some parts of the world.

21 You are called to a stranded cetacean on a beach and start your clinical examination, which is limited to the equipment available in the back of your car. What are the essential components of your examination?

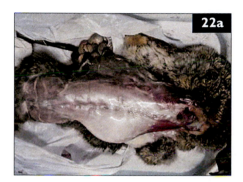

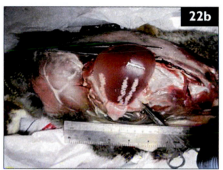

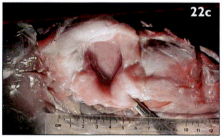

22 A wild rabbit was found dead on permanent sheep pasture. It was in fairly fresh condition, had external signs of myxomatosis and an unusual swelling on the right side. A post-mortem examination was carried out to assess the swelling (22a, b). The site was dissected and the contents removed and identified (22c).
i. What is the structure within the swelling in the musculature of the right back muscles?
ii. Was it likely to have contributed to the rabbit's death?
iii. Is this a common problem?

21

- Determining the species and size of the animal.
- Determining if it is weaned (check its length against known species lengths, presence/absence of vibrissae on the beak/rostrum, presence/absence of lingual papillae and umbilicus).
- Nutritional state/body condition (concavity/convexity of the lumbar muscles adjacent to the dorsal fin).

21 *Blood sampling sites in cetaceans*

Lateral surface of dorsal fin

Ventral surface of tail flukes (N.B. central tail veins also accessible from dorsal surface of flukes)

- Assessing the severity of any trauma.
- Checking for skin peeling/cracking (worsens with time out of water).
- Checking for signs of dehydration (loss of skin/muscle tone).
- Assessing reflexes and jaw/tongue tone.
- Checking for discharges from orifices (including blood).
- Lung auscultation and assessing the character and rate of respirations (porpoises/dolphins normally 2–5 breaths/minute; less in larger cetaceans).
- Assessing for signs of shock (including increasing expiratory–inspiratory gap and capillary refill time).
- Checking temperature (taken with thermistor probe inserted 20–30 cm into rectum depending on size; normal range 36–37.5°C [96.8–99.5°F], >40°C [104°F] critical; >42°C [107.6°F] terminal).
- Where nearby laboratory services are available, analyses of blood samples drawn from the central tail vessels (arteriovenous complexes) in smaller animals and the dorsal fin vessels in larger animals (**21**). Useful parameters include haematocrit, leucogram, muscle enzymes, urea and creatinine. Reference ranges for some species are available.

22 i. *Coenurus serialis*, the larval stage of the adult tapeworm *Taenia serialis*, in which the scolices are typically arranged in serial lines. Distinct rows of white structures can be seen radiating along the surface in **22b**.
ii. The intermediate stages of this tapeworm locate in connective tissue sites. In this rabbit the cyst has developed in the muscles, forming a smooth-walled space, without evidence of sepsis, and causing no compromise to the rabbit's health. Death was due to myxomatosis. In certain locations (e.g. the orbit) the cysts can compromise the rabbit's health.
iii. The adult tapeworms are parasites of dogs and foxes. The pasture where this rabbit was found is dog free and foxes are seen rarely. The parasite cyst can affect rabbits and hares, but it is non-lethal and an uncommon finding.

23 A common buzzard is found dead. It is in an emaciated condition. On post-mortem examination you observe numerous whitish focal lesions in the liver and spleen and nodular swellings on the wall of the gizzard and along the intestines. There is a gross excess of pericardial fluid and a mass of urates in the cloaca (23a).

i. What is your provisional diagnosis?
ii. Which of the lesions are characteristic of the disease, and which are unusual?
iii. What tests would you carry out to investigate this case further?
iv. What other organisms might cause similar lesions?

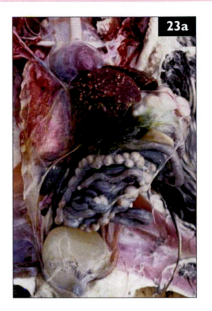

24 A fledgling common blackbird, 'rescued' from an attack by a domesticated cat, is presented with multiple wounds to the body (24). Examination reveals a bird in good body condition with fresh wounds, some of which appear to be skin lacerations, exposing the underlying damaged musculature, but one wound on the lateral body wall has clearly punctured the body cavity.

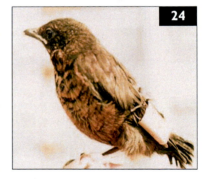

i. What are the main factors to be considered in the assessment of this common situation, and what course of action is appropriate?
ii. Would attempts to treat this bird be of any significant conservation value?

23 i. Avian tuberculosis caused by *Mycobacterium avium* subsp. *avium*.

ii. Focal lesions in both the spleen and liver are commonly seen in avian tuberculosis. However, lesions can occur in any organ. Typically, the lesions consist of caseous pus and are often partly mineralized, which makes them feel gritty when cut. The nodular lesions in the wall of the gizzard and along the

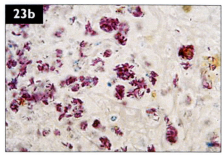

intestine are unusual and probably arose in lymph nodes. Excess fluid in the pericardium and cloaca is commonly seen in birds suffering from chronic debility.

iii. Make impression smears from the cut surface of lesions onto at least three microscope slides. Stain one with Gram and one with Ziehl–Neelsen and examine them with a high-power objective (at least 60x). If you see clumps of acid-fast organisms (**23b**), there is little justification in most cases for further tests. If no acid-fast organisms are seen, check the Gram smear for other organisms and consider submitting tissues for cultural examination. Sections of affected organs could also be examined histopathologically using Gram, ZN and H&E stains.

iv. *Yersinia pseudotuberculosis*, *Salmonella* spp., *Listeria* spp. and *Erysipelothrix* spp. can cause similar focal liver lesions.

24 i. Cat bite wounds are commonly associated with a variety of bacterial infections, frequently leading to fatal septicaemia/toxaemia. The chance of successful treatment (supportive/medical/surgical) in such a severe case is very low and euthanasia might be the most humane approach. The success rate with less severely injured fledglings is also poor, usually due to failure to control infection. Uninjured fledglings are best returned to the site where found and placed in a safe position for their parents to relocate. If this is not possible, they can, with patience, be easily reared by hand.

ii. As with most species of passerine birds, the dynamics of the wild population allow for a high rate of natural loss. A pair of blackbirds in a breeding season might hatch two or three clutches, each averaging five eggs; however, they will only rear to independence an average of two or three offspring, of which 60% will fail to survive the first year. Casualties of displaced fledglings might represent part of this natural loss and attempts to rehabilitate these birds in a species that is under no serious threat is unlikely to be of any real conservation value.

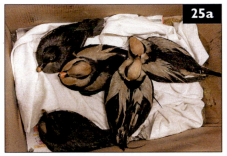

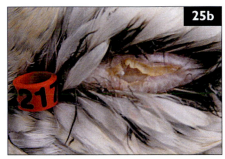

25 Following an oilspill in Northern Europe, several hundred oiled seabirds are brought into a temporary centre for rehabilitation. The predominant species are long-tailed ducks and common goldeneye. For several days they are held in small groups in cardboard boxes, on newspaper and towels as bedding (25a). As facilities are created in the temporary centre, standard rehabilitation techniques for the treatment and washing of oiled birds are followed. The first group of birds is introduced to water. They seem to be waterproof and are bright and responsive. However, the next morning several of the birds are found to be waterlogged and hypothermic, and two are dead in the water. Lesions typical of those found on examination of both dead and live birds are shown (25b).
i. What is the cause of the lesions over the keel bone?
ii. What is the probable cause of the failure of waterproofing?
iii. Can the live birds be treated, and what is the prognosis?
iv. What advice would you give to the rehabilitators?

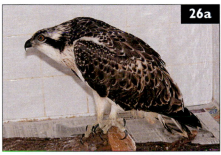

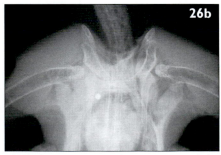

26 An osprey is shown (26a). It had been found on the ground near a trout lake in southern England and was unable to fly. A ventrodorsal radiograph of the bird's pectoral region was taken (26b).
i. What lesions can be seen?
ii. What would be your approach to managing this case?

25 **i.** Pressure necrosis. Even with soft bedding, seabirds are very prone to keel lesions. They can only stand on land for short periods, so spend their time resting on their keel, which rapidly ulcerates.

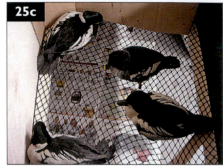

ii. Leaking of serous fluid from the wound onto surrounding feathers. This clogs the feathers and causes them to clump together, making a hole in the waterproof outer layer of feathers. Water then soaks through to the down feathers and the bird becomes waterlogged, loses buoyancy and becomes hypothermic due to lack of insulation and increased heat loss.

iii. Treatments attempted, with limited success, include suturing the lesion with subcuticular sutures and providing a warm water pool to prevent hypothermia. The prognosis is guarded, and is hopeless unless birds can be maintained on water to reduce keel pressure.

iv. Prior to washing, oiled seabirds should be kept in net bottomed cages (**25c**). This minimizes the pressure on the keel bone and feather damage from faeces, which drops through the netting. Birds should be triaged and those showing evidence of keel lesions euthanased. Rehabilitation efforts are concentrated on unaffected birds. Following washing, birds should be maintained on water. A small ledge should be provided for birds to leave the water and avoid drowning if they start to become waterlogged.

26 **i.** A fractured coracoid bone and a round metallic density suggestive of a piece of lead shot are visible.

ii. The coracoid fracture is minimally displaced. This type of fracture often does well with rest. Lead shot does not normally need to be removed from soft tissue unless infection is present. Lead is not significantly absorbed from this particular site, thus preventing heavy metal toxicity. This bird was rested for two weeks in a treatment bay. It then spent a further two months in rehabilitation aviaries, the space allowed being gradually increased as flight improved. It was fed on fresh trout while in captivity. As these birds migrate, release had to be timed to coincide with migration times. It was deemed 'ready' in early autumn to coincide with the osprey's southern migration. A satellite tracking device was fitted and the bird released. After a few days spent on the south coast of England the bird's signal was picked up in northern Spain less than 10 days post release

Post-release monitoring is of vital importance in assessing treatment and rehabilitation success. In this case it could be seen that conservative management gave a favourable outcome and that the bird had, in fact, been fit for release.

27 You are called to a facility where approximately 40 guillemots have been admitted following an oil spill. Pending washing they are housed in a concrete floored barn in pens divided up by bales of hay. Approximately half have already been washed and are on an outdoor covered pool consisting of a concrete-edged, shallow, static fresh water pool with no filtration. They are fed freshly defrosted sprats in the water. Six birds have died within 24 hours of the washing process.
i. What are your differential diagnoses for the cause of death, and how would you proceed to diagnose the problem?
ii. What changes would you make to the facility to improve their success rates?

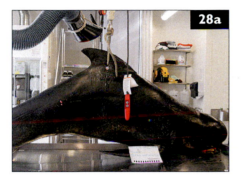

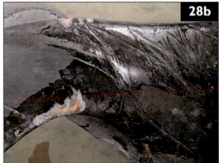

28 A long-finned pilot whale is observed in a harbour on the north-eastern seaboard of the USA. The animal is remaining at the surface, circling in an anticlockwise pattern, with breaths every 1–2 minutes. It is actively avoiding boats and shallow water, and evades attempts by the local strandings network staff to herd it out into deep water. A few days later, attempts to herd

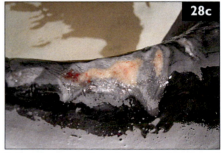

it into deep water are successful, but the following morning the animal is found stranded on a nearby beach. As it is impossible to refloat the animal, it is euthanased and taken to a marine laboratory for necropsy (28a). These lesions are seen on superficial inspection (28b, c).
i. How would you describe the body condition of this animal?
ii. What do you consider to be the cause and time-scale of these lesions, and what impact do you think they may have had on the eventual fate of this animal?

27 i. Fungal infection, maladaption due to either inadequate body condition or incomplete washing. Dead birds should be subjected to post-mortem examination and samples taken for histopathology and bacterial and/or fungal culture. The cause of death in these birds was aspergillosis (27). Remaining live birds are likely to be infected and should be investigated by radiographic and endoscopic examination. Any with grossly evident aspergillosis should be euthanased, and the rest, plus new additions, treated prophylactically with antifungals (e.g. itraconazole).

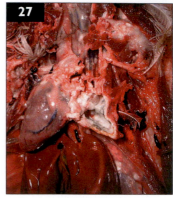

ii. Even in clean environments, fungal spore levels can be sufficient to cause clinical disease. Vegetation, hay or straw results in a very high environmental fungal spore load. Better ventilated, uncontaminated environments should be used and all organic material removed. Unless the birds spend all their time on the water, the concrete floor should be covered with soft matting to avoid foot lesions. The birds should be fed fish in shallow water-filled bowls or trays, separate to the water they swim in, to avoid recontamination of plumage with fish oil. The water should be filtered, or at least be continuously overflowing, and skimmed to avoid recontamination with faeces. Fresh water is commonly used, but salt water is the natural environment of such birds and is preferred.

28 i. This animal is emaciated. The body shape over the lumbar muscles between the midline and the transverse processes of the vertebral column is markedly concave. There is a visible 'neck' behind the blowhole.

ii. There are abrasions on the fluke stock dorsally and laterally and cross-hatched impressions on the peduncle, typical of rope abrasions from entanglement. Cetaceans can often free themselves of entanglements over time and many show typical scars. On the eastern seaboard of the USA there is a significant problem with entanglement of large whales (and seals and marine turtles) in the vertical lines of lobster pots. However, this is not the only cause, and entanglement in set nets (drift nets or bottom tangle nets) or moving trawl nets usually leads to death (termed fishery bycatch).

There is evidence of healing, which suggests that the wounds are more than a few days old; however, the depth of the lesions does not necessarily suggest that the entanglement was prolonged over weeks or months. It is difficult to attribute the emaciated condition of this animal solely to the effects of entanglement, although it may have been a contributory factor. Other potential causes for the emaciated condition of this animal should be investigated by a full necropsy.

29 A Canada goose weighing 2.4 kg is presented to your clinic. The goose has been living in a park by the same pond for three years and local residents feed it bread, crackers or popcorn on a daily basis. About a week and a half ago they noticed that the goose's voice was changing. A few days ago they noticed that it had green diarrhoea, and today the goose did not stand when approached. It was generally depressed and weak; respiration was normal; there was a ruffled appearance to the neck and head feathers and lice were present; the eyes were dull; the mouth and nares were normal; and the goose could use its legs but was in a sternal position. PCV was 0.29 l/l (29%), buffy coat was 1% and total solids were 1.8 g/dl. A dorso-ventral radiograph was taken (**29a**).

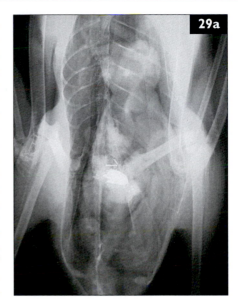

i. What additional diagnostic test(s) would you run?
ii. What conditions are on your differential list, and which is/are highest?
iii. Provide a stabilization and treatment plan for this bird.

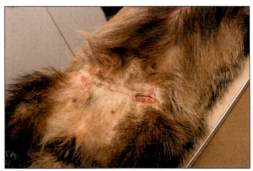

30 i. What does this image show (**30**), and how is the injury likely to have been sustained?
ii. What would be your approach and considerations when treating such injuries?

29 i. Submit a blood sample for heavy metals (minimum lead and zinc).

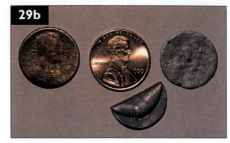

ii. Crop impaction: possible lead or other heavy metal poisoning; possible foreign body blockage; possible soybean toxicity, possible trauma. Density in ventriculus: foreign body ingestion, most likely lead or zinc. An elevated zinc blood level (80 ppm [>40 ppm is toxic]) confirmed a diagnosis of heavy metal toxicity. Pennies minted in the USA after 1981 contain up to 98% zinc, coated with copper (29b).

iii. 2.5% dextrose in lactated Ringer's solution (D2.5LRS) should be given i/v and repeated q12h for 24 hours. D2.5LRS or another oral rehydrating solution should be given. There should be access to water but no other food (especially avoid any solids like corn or pelleted feeds that might further grind the metallic objects). Pyrethrin powder is applied to treat the lice. Once stable, the treatment for lead and zinc poisoning is the same (i.e. administration of a chelating agent such as calcium EDTA or Succimer and removal of any metal still visible in the GI tract). In this goose the penny can be removed through endoscopy, gastric lavage or by surgical ventriculotomy.

30 i. A deep cutaneous circumferential linear wound around the ventral caudal abdomen of a badger. This was caused by a wire snare.

ii. The badger should be sedated and fully examined. Concurrent injuries to the limbs and jaw are common, associated with the animal's attempts to escape from the snare. Where wounds extend into deeper structures or there are concurrent injuries, the chance of successful release is poor and euthanasia is recommended. Where the wounds are limited to the cutaneous and subcutaneous structures, they should be cleaned, débrided and, where appropriate, sutured. Open wound management includes daily flushing with saline or dilute chlorhexidine solution and the application of topical hydrogel products to encourage granulation and epithelialization. Wounds suitable for suturing are those that are gaping, but have clean viable subcutaneous tissue, and skin edges that can be closed without tension. If there is any uncertainty regarding tissue viability, open wound management should continue for a few days and the wound be reassessed. Ischaemic damage from the snare may result in a delay in tissue necrosis of several days. Animals that have been snared should be kept under observation for at least one week, even where initially wound healing appears to be progressing well. Broad-spectrum antibiotics, fluid therapy and analgesics should be implemented as appropriate.

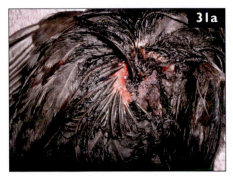

31 You are presented with a blackbird that has been found in a client's garden and brought indoors by her cat. It has a puncture wound near the shoulder (**31a**) and is unable to fly.
i. Is this wound likely to be a cat bite wound? If not, what is the most likely aetiology, and why?
ii. What would be the most useful diagnostic procedure?
iii. What is the likely prognosis, and what action might you take?

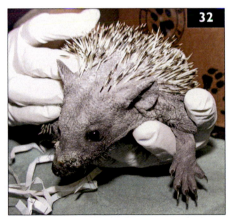

32 You are presented with this hedgehog (**32**) in late summer. What considerations would you make in your triage and decision making regarding this case?

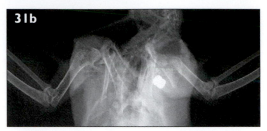

31 i. Although cat bites are an extremely common source of morbidity and mortality in wild passerines, this wound has the classical appearance of a ballistic entry wound. The feathers entering the hole are drawn in by the pressure wave preceding a shotgun or airgun pellet.

ii. Radiographic evaluation is vital in any case of ballistic injury or suspected predator trauma. This radiograph (31b), showing a fracture of the humerus and an associated airgun pellet, was obtained at post-mortem examination from a similar case involving a wood pigeon.

iii. The injury noted in the radiograph, if the result of blunt impact trauma, would have a very poor prognosis for full return to flight and subsequent release. Because the injury is associated with an area of soft tissue damage extending from the entry point to a depth unknown, and because of the presence of not only the pellet, but also indrawn skin and feather material, the likelihood of infection and fibrosis is even greater and the prognosis grim. Euthanasia is the preferred outcome.

32 Hedgehogs hibernate over winter and this affects the release of underweight (<550 g) juveniles in the winter months. The hedgehog illustrated is a juvenile and underweight for its size. There is evidence of chronic skin disease: generalized hair loss, hyperkeratosis (especially around the pinnae and rostrum) and paucity of spines. There are no acute clinical signs requiring first aid treatment. The hedgehog should be fully examined and a diagnosis of the skin condition made using suitable diagnostic tests (e.g. skin scrape for parasites, fungal culture).

The main considerations are the chronicity of the skin problem and the likely time for it to resolve with correct treatment. This, together with the age of the hedgehog and the time of year, means that a protracted time in captivity may be required. There are costs attached to both the diagnostic procedures and the drugs. Ultimately, the hedgehog will need a suitable release site away from main roads. The likely causes of the skin problem (mites or ringworm) are common in the hedgehog population.

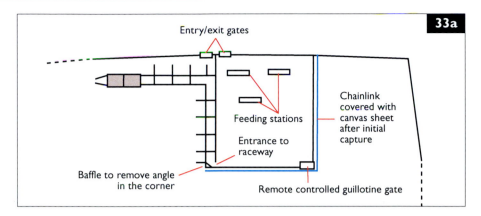

33a

Entry/exit gates

Feeding stations

Chainlink covered with canvas sheet after initial capture

Entrance to raceway

Baffle to remove angle in the corner

Remote controlled guillotine gate

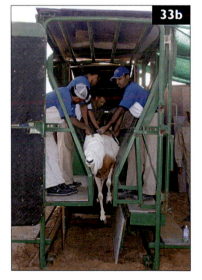

33b

33 The equipment illustrated (**33a, b**) is used to physically restrain animals from a herd of semi-free-ranging scimitar-horned oryx inhabiting a large desert reserve area for annual vaccinations, hoof trimming and health checks, including blood sampling. Describe briefly the main elements of the system, including how the animals might be moved into the capture system?

34 i. What are the advantages of using physical restraint compared with chemical restraint when dealing with groups of ungulates?
ii. What problems can occur during the physical restraint of large ungulates?

33 Animals are first habituated to being fed in an enclosed feeding area out of which a raceway leads to where the restraint equipment is set up. The feeding area should only have one entry/exit gate in operation during the capture habituation. The gate is closed manually or automatically (remote controlled guillotine gate) after the animals have entered the feeding area. Utilizing feeding stations and installing the raceway in advance of the catch conditions animals to changes in their surroundings. After the gate is closed, a coloured canvas sheet is suspended on the outside of the chain link fence. Other canvas sheets are then used within the feeding pen to encourage the animals into the raceway, where animals are quickly split into small groups (2–3) using sliding doors to avoid injury or aggression. From these groups, individuals are moved up a ramp and restrained using a V-shaped drop floor Junior Tamer or larger Tamer 2 unit. The raceway system is modular and, along with the Tamer unit, can be transported readily between sites.

34 **i.** Chemical restraint techniques are useful for the rapid induction of anaesthesia/sedation of individual animals, but is not practical for handling large numbers. Mobile raceway and restraint equipment (see **33**) gives the flexibility to move many animals safely, with repeat treatment and manipulation of animals as necessary. The raceway system enables an animal to be restrained every 5–10 minutes, thus processing up to 50 medium-sized ungulates a day. The equipment can be mobilized and moved between sites easily.
ii. Physical restraint can affect blood parameters and often results in muscle and liver enzymes being acutely elevated, possibly due to capture stress. Medical problems that can occur include:
- Capture myopathy.
- Asphyxiation. If an animal is dropped in the unit after being left with access to food for too long in the feeding pen before being moved into the raceway, its weight on a fully engorged stomach can cause regurgitation of rumen contents (and asphyxiation). Food should only be used in small amounts as an incentive to get the animals into the pen.
- Trauma. Minor abrasions, scuffing and horn injuries can occur to animals within the Tamer and raceway system. These are usually superficial and easily treated.
- Late-term abortion. Heavily pregnant animals should not be dropped in the unit.

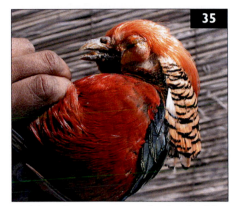

35 This free-ranging golden pheasant was submitted with an ocular discharge, a persistent cough and a swollen head (35). Other pheasants in the flock were similarly affected.
i. List the diseases that can cause these clinical signs in gamebirds.
ii. What is the most likely diagnosis, and how would you confirm it?
iii. What age group is most susceptible to infection?
iv. What are the features of the disease that lead to mortality?
v. What treatment should be given to the flock?
vi. What control measures are important?

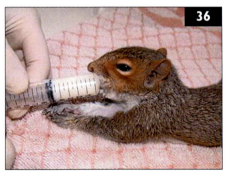

36 Many requests for veterinary advice and assistance concern abandoned or orphaned young birds and mammals, such as the animal seen in this picture (36).
i. What is this species?
ii. In the UK, what legal and ethical issues should be considered when presented with such a patient?

35 i. Syngamiasis, mycoplasmosis, chlamydophilosis, cryptosporidiosis, Newcastle disease, infectious laryngotracheitis, infectious bronchitis.

ii. Sinusitis caused by *Mycoplasma gallisepticum*. Diagnosis is based on culture of swabs taken from the trachea, conjunctiva, choanal cleft or sinus (using special culture media). Mycoplasmosis can be confirmed indirectly using serology. A positive serological test result plus a suspicious history and clinical signs allow a presumptive diagnosis to be made. Molecular techniques such as species-specific DNA probes or PCR are also useful.

iii. Chicks 2–8 weeks of age.

iv. Mortality depends on secondary factors such as concurrent infection (e.g. *Chlamydophila* or *Pasteurella* spp.). The eyes are affected first, resulting in photophobia, swelling of the eyelids, watery discharge, blepharoconjunctivitis and keratitis. Death results from starvation.

v. Antimycoplasma drugs, including tiamulin, tylosin, spiramycin and enrofloxacin, in the drinking water.

vi. Mycoplasmosis can be transmitted vertically via the egg and horizontally through direct contact or aerosol droplets via the respiratory tract, especially at times of stress. *M. gallisepticum* can exist for short periods of time on dust, litter, feathers and rubber boots. Contaminated litter (e.g. from poultry farms) may pose a risk to free-living birds. Strategic in-feed medication of adults during times of stress (e.g. when birds are moved) may help reduce spread. Contact with wild birds, which can be reservoirs for *Mycoplasma* infection, should be avoided.

36 i. A juvenile grey squirrel.

ii. An immature wild animal is often assumed to be orphaned or abandoned, but this is rarely the case and animals are often taken into care unnecessarily. Unless the parents are known to have been killed or injured, in most cases the patient has matured to the point where it can leave the safety of its nest and start exploring its environment. These immature individuals are often unable to fly or fend for themselves and rely on staying hidden in order to avoid predators. Their parents will continue to feed their young, but will not approach unless it is safe for them to do so; therefore, they are mistakenly thought to have been abandoned or orphaned.

In the UK, non-indigenous birds and mammals cannot legally be released into the wild under the Wildlife and Countryside Act (1981), which contains measures for preventing the establishment of non-native species that may be detrimental to native wildlife. The release of animals and planting of plants listed in Schedule 9 of the Act is prohibited. The grey squirrel is listed in Schedule 9 and so it is illegal for grey squirrels to be released into the wild. This should be borne in mind when a grey squirrel is presented for rehabilitation.

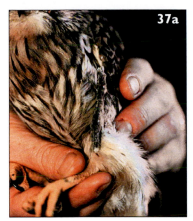

37 i. What type of fracture fixation system has been used to stabilize the tibial fracture in this kestrel (37a)?
ii. What are the advantages and disadvantages of this method?

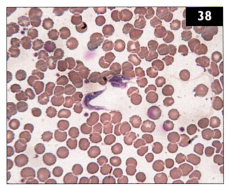

38 This photomicrograph (38) is of a blood smear stained with a Romanowsky-type stain (Speedy-Diff™). The blood sample was taken under general anaesthesia from a two-year-old male badger in May as part of a badger capture–mark–recapture study in the UK. The badger was in good body condition.
i. What is the microparasite in the centre of the photograph.
ii. What are the possible consequences of infection?

37 i. A bilateral uniplanar external skeletal fixator system using hypodermic needles as full pins and a thermosetting plastic material (methylmethacrylate) to form the lateral and medial bars.

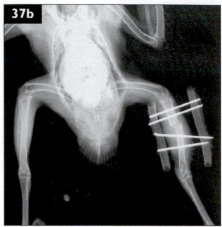

ii. This method of fixation produces good fracture site stability, does not immobilize the proximal and distal joints and allows rapid return to normal use of the limb. There is minimal soft tissue damage. Pins run medial to lateral, so minimizing any potential damage to the distal tendons of insertion of the cranial tibial and long digital extensor muscles. Rotation at the fracture site is limited. The medullary cavity is not broached, making the technique especially suitable for compound fractures. Fixators are light, inexpensive and easily removed, and usually well tolerated. The main disadvantage is the risk to nerves and blood vessels crossing the craniolateral aspect of the tibia. Great care must be taken placing the pins. Intramedullary pinning of the tibia using a medial approach to the limb is the preferred technique. It is not always possible to obtain perfect alignment using an external fixator (**37b**). Pin fracture or loosening is not a significant issue in birds because they are lighter and fracture healing is more rapid. The acrylic resin used in this example has a very strong odour, may burn the skin and takes a long time to set. More user-friendly acrylic products are available (e.g. bone cement, dental acrylic).

38 i. Based on the morphological appearance, the parasite is a trypanosome and, from previous reports, it is likely to be *Trypanosoma (Megatrypanum) pestanai.*
ii. Low and intermittent levels of parasitaemia associated with trypanosome infections mean diagnosis by this method is likely to underestimate the prevalence of infection. Megatrypanosomes are not generally associated with clinical signs, but the occurrence of pathogenic effects and/or the degree to which badgers may be trypanotolerant are currently unknown. Pathogenic effects might include anaemia, generalized lymphadenomegaly, pyrexia associated with a parasitaemia and progressive condition loss. The vector for *T. pestanai* is also currently unknown, but possible candidates include the badger flea *Paraceras melis* and tabanid biting flies.

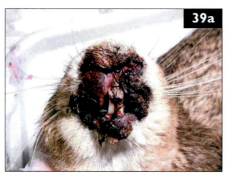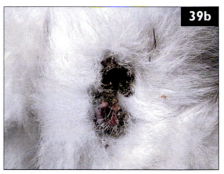

39 An immature male hare was found lying down dying at pasture and was euthanased by neck dislocation and submitted for post-mortem examination shortly afterwards. Severe crusting and dermatitis were evident on the face around the mouth and nostrils and several pustules were present inside the lips (39a). Similar dermatitis was noted in the perineal region around the anus and sheath (39b). There was absence of internal fat reserves and only 17 g of food in the stomach: the alimentary tract was unremarkable. No diarrhoea or internal coccidial lesions were present. The spleen was massively enlarged: adrenals and kidneys were also swollen. A swab from heart blood was sterile.
i. What is the most likely cause of the skin lesions?
ii. What is the most likely cause of the weight loss and prostration?

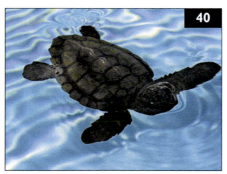

40 What are the husbandry requirements for loggerhead sea turtle hatchlings (40) kept in captivity for a head-starting programme, and what parameters must be maintained as a constant?

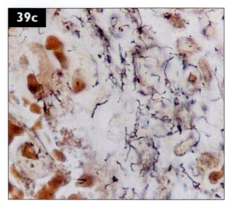

39 i. Hare syphilis. Bosma-Steiner silver staining of a facial skin histology section reveals *Treponema cuniculi* spirochaetes (39c). The condition is sexually transmitted and is quite common; however, it is not usually so severe and is not usually associated with death. Rabbits also are susceptible.
ii. The swollen spleen and histological appearance of the spleen, adrenal glands and kidneys confirmed severe secondary amyloidosis. This was presumably in response to the chronically infected skin lesions. The kidneys were particularly badly affected in this case, so the severe illness may have reflected renal failure.

40 Loggerhead hatchlings are especially sensitive to water salinity (they require sea water) and ambient water temperature (requiring a temperature range between 26 and 28°C in the first stages). These parameters need to be maintained constantly throughout the captivity period. The use of ultraviolet light is also important to ensure adequate vitamin D synthesis and, therefore, correct calcium metabolism. There is a lack of knowledge concerning what these animals eat in the wild during their juvenile stages. Therefore, as wide as possible a range of different foods should be given. Recipes for home-made, gel-based diets have been published, and a mixture of different fish, crustaceans and molluscs, dusted with a commercially available calcium powder, has also been used successfully. This is preferred, especially in the last stages before the animals are released, so that they get used to their natural food in the wild. Commercially available gels for carnivorous marine animals can also be used to balance this diet.

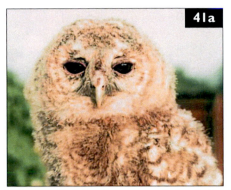

41 A tawny owl chick close to fledging is presented after being found on the ground in a local wood (**41a**). The bird appears to be in good condition with no obvious injuries. The finders are asking for advice, as they are keen to keep the bird and rear it by hand.

i. What are the main problems associated with hand-rearing a young bird such as this, and what advice should be given?

ii. Very often, in cases like this, the bird has been in captivity for several days, or longer, and the site where the bird was first located is not known. What are the options for handling and releasing young tawny owls in these circumstances?

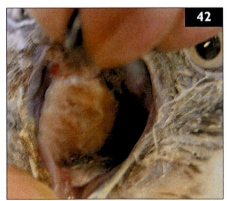

42 A thin debilitated northern sparrowhawk is presented with this lesion in the mouth (**42**).

i. What are the likely differential diagnoses?

ii. How should these be distinguished?

iii. How would you treat/manage this condition?

41 i. Inappropriate diet and social and sexual imprinting on human handlers. Osteodystrophy is a common problem in hand-reared owls (**41b**). Imprinting on handlers can result in birds that have no fear of humans and could, during the breeding season, recognize humans entering their territory as being conspecific invaders and attack. To prevent imprinting, the amount of visual and auditory contact with humans must be kept to a minimum and contact with conspecific individuals encouraged. Due to these problems, the best advice is to attempt to return the bird to where it was found, where it is very likely to be reunited with its parents.

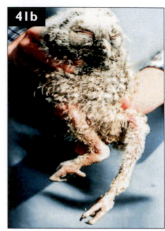

ii. With help from a local naturalist, the chick might be fostered by placing it in a tawny owl nest with young of a similar age. Failing this, the bird should be passed to a rehabilitation unit with the facilities and experience in handling and releasing young tawny owls. The timing of release of juveniles of any species requires knowledge of their natural history. If none of these options are available, euthanasia could be considered.

42 i. Trichomonosis ('frounce'), candidiasis, bacterial infection (especially secondary to trauma), capillariasis.
ii. Wet preparations and Gram-stained and trichrome (e.g. Diff Quik®)-stained preparations of crust and underlying mucous membranes should be examined. In this case there were many motile protozoans present, and stains of the crust showed a heavy mixed bacterial load with associated inflammatory cells. A diagnosis of trichomonosis with secondary bacterial infection was made.
iii. The bird was given metronidazole (50 mg/kg p/o q24h) and clavulanate–amoxicillin (150 mg/kg p/o q12h) for five days. The oral lesion was cleaned twice a day with dilute povidone–iodine before the bird was tube fed with Critical Care Formula® (Vetark). Trichomonosis is generally contracted from eating infected pigeons. Most accipiters show good immunity to the disease unless there is prior trauma or they are immunocompromised. In this case the bird was relatively young and had a heavy intestinal endoparasite load. This illustrates the need always to assess for any underlying disease as well as the obvious clinical lesions.

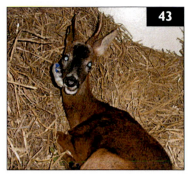

43 This deer (43) was hit by a car and fractured its mandible. It was repaired using an external fixator.
i. What species of deer is this?
ii. Are there any welfare issues to be considered in this case?
iii. What are the risks associated with general anaesthesia in deer?

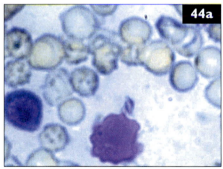
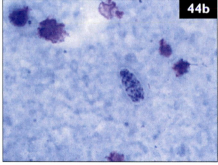

44 Two out of a group of eight Bennett's wallabies have died in three days, another is showing neurological signs, falling over repeatedly, and a fourth has laboured breathing. Gross post-mortem examination of the dead wallabies shows congested lungs and enlarged, mottled mesenteric lymph nodes. Romanowsky-stained impression smears from the heart of one of the animals are shown (44a, b).
i. What is the likely cause of these animals' illness?
ii. What further tests could be carried out to confirm this diagnosis?
iii. How can this condition be treated?
iv. How can it be prevented in the future?
v. What other species are highly susceptible to this disease?

43 i. Roe deer.

ii. Generally, wild deer do not cope well with confinement. They have to be kept very quiet, away from people and other disturbances. If hospitalized, they should be in a purposely adapted building, such as a shed with no windows, but good ventilation. Care must be taken with opening any doors, as deer may try to jump towards the light. If treatment is likely to last more than two weeks, careful consideration should given as to whether euthanasia is the most humane option. The deer illustrated here was kept in a purpose-built mammal shed at a wildlife hospital and successfully released six weeks later.

iii. Deer can suffer from capture myopathy, so should be manually restrained or chased as little as possible. They are ruminants, so great care must be taken to ensure that rumen contents are not aspirated under general anaesthesia. The head should be elevated and ideally the deer should be kept in sternal recumbancy. If lateral recumbancy is necessary, it is preferable to lie the animal on its right side. Profuse salivation is common, as the swallowing reflex disappears early, therefore intubation is generally recommended.

44 i. Toxoplasmosis. Two *Toxoplasma gondii* tachyzoites (**44a**) and a tissue cyst (**44b**) are demonstrated.

ii. Immunohistochemical staining of tissue sections.

iii. Pyrimethamine (0.5 mg/kg p/o q24h) plus sulphadiazine (60 mg/kg p/o q24h in 3–4 divided doses) plus folic acid supplementation (1 mg/kg q24h); or clindamycin (11 mg/kg p/o or i/m q12h for at least 30 days); or spiramycin (3 g per 70 kg daily p/o in divided doses); or atovaquone (100 mg/kg p/o q2h4). The rest of the group may be treated with trimethoprim/sulphonamide in the food. The food trough should be thoroughly cleaned and any hay removed and replaced with a fresh batch.

iv. The definitive hosts are cats, and the usual source of infection for herbivores is oocysts in cat faeces. Cats should be kept out of feed stores and, if possible, out of hay barns. If cats are kept for rodent control, adult, neutered cats that are already seropositive for *T. gondii* should be kept, since shedding of oocysts is greatest on first infection. Once wallabies are infected, the protozoa remain in the tissues lifelong and infection may be reactivated by stress. Wallabies should be treated prophylactically with oral sulphadiazine if they are moved to another enclosure.

v. Australian marsupials, lemurs, marmosets and tamarins and the European brown hare, as well as Pallas cats.

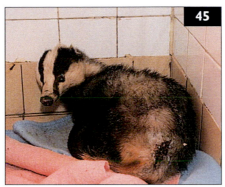

45 What criteria need to be considered when releasing an adult badger back into the wild following treatment for territorial fight wound injuries (**45**)?

46 A 21-day-old stone curlew chick in a mixed species avicultural unit presented with severe dyspnoea and a mucoid ocular and nasal discharge (**46**). A blacksmith plover at the same unit had died suddenly the previous night and had been submitted for post-mortem examination, but no results were available. A number of other white-bellied bustard chicks were also observed with mild respiratory signs, decreased food consumption and general lethargy. The building was situated adjacent to lakes, which accommodated large numbers of both pinioned and free-flying waterfowl. Older chicks from the rearing unit, including the dead

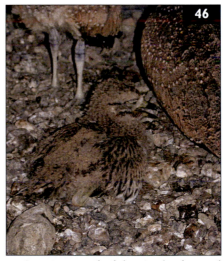

blacksmith plover, had been housed outdoors in pens near the lakes in the day and brought into the rearing unit at night. Over the course of one week a further three birds died in the rearing unit after presenting with respiratory signs.

i. What diagnostic tests are available to investigate respiratory tract disease in these birds?

ii. List the differential diagnoses for respiratory tract signs in birds.

45 Is it fit and in good body condition? A casualty badger with territorial wounds is sometimes an elderly animal that is no longer a viable clan member and is simply cast out by the other badgers. This type of casualty should not be released and should be euthanased. A fit badger should be returned to the area it was found in. Territorial wounding is caused during clan member disputes over food, sett choices and right to mate. A badger with a territorial fight wound will know where it stands within the pecking order of its clan. If released into another badger clan area, it will not be familiar with sett locations, feeding areas or have any status within the group. It will probably be treated as an alien and chased away.

The time of year is important. There are peak times of territorial activity amongst badgers, notably February to May and October to December (in the northern hemisphere). If a badger has to be released into an alien area, this should be done outside of these periods.

46 i.
• Aerobic bacterial and fungal culture on conjunctival and nasal–choanal swabs.
• *Chlamydophila* testing.
• Cytology on samples of nasal and ocular discharges.
• Virus isolation on swabs of the ocular and nasal discharge and pooled cloacal–choanal swabs. For avian influenza virus the standard is to use 9–14-day-old embryonating chicken eggs.
• *Mycoplasma* culture on swabs collected from the ocular and nasal discharge and the trachea.
• Rapid antigen testing on faecal samples for avian influenza, Newcastle disease and *Chlamydophila*.
• Collection and storage of sera to allow for the demonstration of seroconversion using acute and convalescent serum samples against any isolated agent.
ii. Differential diagnoses include:
• Bacterial infections, in particular *Pseudomonas aeruginosa*, *Proteus mirabilis*, *Escherichia coli*, *Klebsiella* spp., *Staphylococcus aureus* and *Mycoplasma* spp.
• Chlamydophilosis.
• Viral infections including paramyxovirus, avipox and avian influenza virus.
• Parasitic infections such as trichomonosis and gapeworm.
• Fungal infections with *Aspergillus* spp. and *Candida albicans*.
• Non-infectious diseases including nasal plugs, irritation of the respiratory tract with dust, toxins or foreign bodies, subcutaneous emphysema or haemorrhage, trauma, neoplasia and space-occupying masses or fluid in the coelomic cavity.
Influenza virus subtype H9N2 was isolated from clinical specimens collected from the live birds and from the tissues of the dead blacksmith plover.

47 An outbreak of avian influenza H9N2 has been diagnosed in an aviculture unit (see **46**).
i. What are the implications for the staff of the aviculture unit?
ii. What treatment or preventive measures can be recommended?

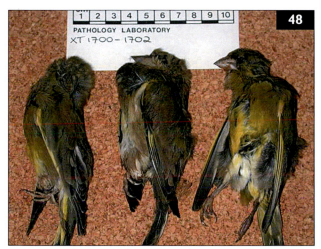

48 A client is concerned after finding three dead greenfinches (**48**) in the garden over the course of a week and has recently seen listless, fluffed-up birds at the garden bird feeding station.
i. What are the most likely causes of the problem?
ii. What advice would you offer?

47 i. Humans can be infected with both low pathogenic (LP) and high pathogenic (HP) avian influenza infections (AIVs). Human illness due to LP AIVs can range from mild symptoms (e.g. conjunctivitis) to generalized influenza-like illness. Human infections have been linked to exposure to infected commercial poultry, and to date (2008) there has not been a documented case of direct transmission of AIVs from a wild bird to a human.

ii. Wild waterfowl are reservoirs for all known HA and NA subtypes of influenza A viruses. The wild waterfowl were suspected to be the source of the outbreak in this example. The transmission of AIV from wild birds to captive birds may be prevented through implementation of good biosecurity measures and the prevention of direct or indirect contact with infected wild birds. Captive birds can also be protected through vaccination using commercially available AIV vaccines. Treatment of individual avian cases of LP AIV using osetamivir phosphate (Tamiflu®) (10 mg/kg p/o q12h) has been reported.

48 i. Infectious disease is the most likely cause. Salmonellosis typically affects gregarious seed-eating species (e.g. greenfinches, house sparrows). Mortality usually occurs during the winter months; transmission is via the faeco-oral route. *Salmonella typhimurium* DT40 and DT56 are the typical causative agents and wild bird populations are believed to act as reservoirs of infection. Lesion predilection sites include the upper alimentary tract, liver and spleen. Salmonellosis is an emerging infectious disease of British finches. Epidemic mortality has occurred yearly since 2005, peaking in the early autumn months, although cases have been recorded throughout the calendar year. Necrotic ingluvitis is associated with this infection. Transmission is direct between birds during the breeding season, or where fresh saliva contaminates shared food or drinking water.

ii. Best practice for garden bird feeding should be followed (e.g. regular cleaning of feeders and tables, provision of fresh food from accredited aflatoxin-free sources, rotation of feeding sites). In the event of a disease outbreak, disinfection measures should be practised and temporary reduction or cessation of feeding considered to discourage congregation of mixed garden bird species at high densities. The client should be advised to follow sensible hygiene precautions because of potential public health implications. There is a risk of cats becoming ill following predation on garden birds affected by salmonellosis.

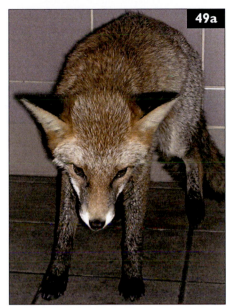

49 This red fox (**49a**) is presented for treatment.
i. What zoonotic diseases may foxes carry?
ii. What preventive measures can be taken to reduce the risks to staff dealing with foxes?

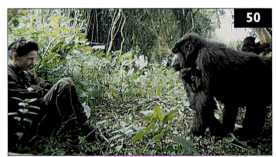

50 Ecotourism is viewed by many as an important conservation tool and a number of free-ranging great ape populations have been habituated to humans for this purpose. However, why is the close contact between humans and mountain gorillas illustrated (**50**) a concern for the conservation of great apes?

49 i. Sarcoptic mange, ringworm. Where rabies is endemic, foxes are often a reservoir host. Several bacterial infections, particularly those causing enteric disease, are zoonotic (e.g. *Campylobacter jejuni*, *Salmonella* spp., coliform infections). Other organisms that may be transmitted in faeces include *Cryptosporidium parvum*, *Giardia* spp., *Toxoplasma*, *Echinococcus granulosus* and *E. multilocularis*. Foxes may also be

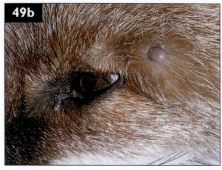

a source of tuberculosis and leptospirosis. Bite wounds from foxes commonly become infected (e.g. with *Streptococcus* spp.). This fox had ticks attached to its skin (**49b**). Ticks may transmit several diseases (e.g. Lyme disease, Q fever, rickettsial disease). Less common zoonotic infections include capillariasis. Where the intermediate agent (sandfly) is present, *Leishmania infantum* may be transmitted from foxes to humans.

ii. Contact with skin, urine, faeces and secretions may spread zoonotic disease. Good hygiene is therefore paramount when examining and treating foxes, including disinfection of holding facilities (to reduce transmission to humans as well as other animals). Latex or nitrile gloves should always be worn when treating wild foxes. Protective equipment such as facemasks, eye goggles and aprons is also useful. In areas where rabies is endemic, staff should be vaccinated and animals handled appropriately to avoid being bitten.

50 Great apes are especially vulnerable to human diseases due to a close taxonomic relationship, and there are increasing reports of human-associated diseases in great ape populations. These include gastrointestinal parasites and sarcoptic mange in mountain gorillas and human paramyxoviruses causing respiratory disease and death in chimpanzees. Consequently, human diseases are considered one of the most serious threats to the survival of great ape populations.

Ecotourism is an important conservation tool, and the habituation of great apes for the purposes of viewing by tourists provides economic incentives to conserve such populations and is a viable strategy for sustainable development. However, due to the potential detrimental impact on great ape populations from the introduction of human diseases, most tourist sites have strict disease prevention regulations. These include stipulating the distance that must be maintained between tourists and great apes, limiting the number of visitors, limiting the length of visits and denying sick tourists access to the great apes, among other measures.

51 A mute swan cygnet with a history of progressive weakness before it died is submitted by a wildlife rehabilitation centre for post-mortem examination. The bird is in an emaciated condition and there are unusual lesions in the thoracic cavity (**51a**).

i. What are the white structures?
ii. What is the most likely diagnosis?
iii. How would you confirm this?
iv. What are the predisposing factors?

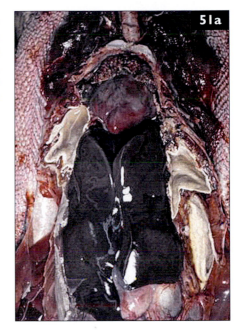

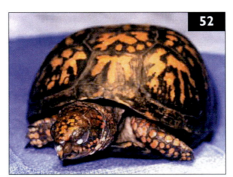

52 This eastern box turtle (**52**) presented to a wildlife rehabilitation facility.
i. Describe the clinical signs noted.
ii. What is a potential infectious aetiology?
iii. How may this be diagnosed?

51 i. Thoracic air sacs. They are greatly thickened and are lined by a thick white deposit.

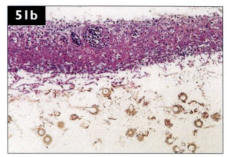

ii. Aspergillosis caused by infection with the fungus *Aspergillus fumigatus*.

iii. As a rapid test, take a small scraping of the white material and place it in a drop of water on a microscope slide. Add a coverslip and examine with a compound microscope with the condenser lowered. Fungal hyphae and/or sporangia confirm a mycotic infection. For definitive diagnosis a sample of air sac lining should be collected aseptically and submitted for cultural examination. Histopathological examination is helpful in some cases. The hyphae stain well by PAS, but the sporangia do not retain stain (51b).

iv. Aspergillosis is often seen in debilitated birds or birds that have been housed on damp hay or straw bedding. It is also a common secondary infection in swans affected by chronic lead poisoning or avian tuberculosis.

52 i. There is a mucopurulent discharge from the nares and eyes, palpebral oedema and depression. This is likely to be a clinical case of mycoplasmosis, but other potential infectious causes include chelonian herpesvirus or iridovirus infection, other bacterial infection including mycobacterioisis, and fungal infection. Other clinical signs typically associated with mycoplasmosis include conjunctivitis, eyes recessed in the sockets and dullness to the scales and scutes.

ii. Tortoise mycoplasmosis was first reported in desert tortoises from the southwestern USA and California and has been associated with dramatic population-level declines of this species. The aetiological agent in desert tortoises is *Mycoplasma agassizii*, which has also been isolated from gopher tortoises from Florida displaying similar clinical signs. Recently, a novel but related *Mycoplasma* species was identified using a PCR assay in box turtles displaying clinical signs consistent with mycoplasmosis. Infection is usually chronic and can often be subclinical. Expression of clinical signs is often intermittent or cyclical and may be associated with stress. A carrier status exists, therefore infected individuals should not be released into the wild.

iii. By culture, although these are fastidious organisms and require special techniques to isolate successfully. PCR assay has proven to be a useful technique to detect the presence of the organism in infected animals.

53 A great horned owl presents to a US wildlife rehabilitation facility displaying dehydration, emaciation, depression, inability to fly, ataxia, a head tremor and head incoordination. A venous blood sample is collected for routine haematology and the results below were obtained. Describe the clinical pathology, and suggest a likely viral diagnosis.

	Results	Reference intervals (ISIS)
PCV	0.28 l/l (28%)	0.3–0.53 (30–53)
WBCs	69.8 × 10^9/l (69.8 × 10^3/µl)	2.89–61.5
Heterophils	46.7 × 10^9/l (46.7 × 10^3/µl	0.86–44.3
Lymphocytes	6.2 × 10^9/l (6.2 × 10^3/µl)	0.07–16.6
Monocytes	6.6 × 10^9/l (6.6 × 10^3/µl)	0.07–5.0
Eosinophils	8.6 × 10^9/l (8.6 × 10^3/µl)	0.06–9.84
Basophils	0.5 × 10^9/l (0.5 × 10^3/µl)	Not available
Band cells	2.3 × 10^9/l (2.3 × 10^3/µl)	Not available

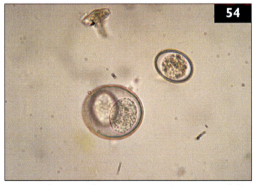

54 This photomicropraph (54) shows material recovered from a badger faecal sample, following flotation in saturated salt solution. The sample was collected from a male badger cub in mid August as part of a badger capture–mark–recapture study in the UK. The cub was approximately six months old and in good body condition.
i. Describe the findings from the faecal flotation.
ii. Briefly discuss implications for the individual cub.

53 Haematology reveals anaemia and a leucocytosis with a heterophilia, eosinophilia, monocytosis and probable left shift. This bird is probably infected with West Nile virus, a flavivirus that was introduced into New York in 1999 and has subsequently spread throughout North America with the exception of Alaska. It is transmitted by mosquitoes, primarily *Culex* species. In addition, direct transmission between birds has been documented under experimental conditions. Most, if not all, North American species of birds are susceptible to infection; however, susceptibility to disease and mortality rates vary depending on the species. American corvid species, including American crows and blue jays, appear to be very susceptible, with high mortality rates, as well as some species of raptors including great horned owls and red-tailed hawks. Sage grouse also appear to have close to a 100% mortality rate.

Infections have been reported in a number of mammalian species of wildlife including fox squirrels, grey squirrels, eastern chipmunks, deer and several species of bats. Additionally, infection has also been reported in American alligators.

54 i. Two species of coccidian oocyst are shown. Based on morphological appearance and previous reports, the smaller oocyst is likely to be *Eimeria melis*, and the larger one a sporulated oocyst of *Isospora melis*.
ii. The implications for the individual cub depend on the intensity of infection, the pathogenicity of the parasite in question and the host's general health and immune status. It is possible to make a quantitative assessment of the parasite burden using a modified McMaster technique, but the practical limitations of this approach, together with circadian variations in oocyst output and the possible occurrence of pathology prior to oocyst production, must all be considered. The relative pathogenicity of these species has not been fully elucidated, but there is some evidence to support mortality and/or impaired growth in cubs associated with *Eimeria melis* infection. In this case the cub was in good body condition, with no evidence of diarrhoea. In addition, it was subsequently recaptured twice in the same year and found to be in good body condition.

55 After some wet weather in the autumn, gamekeepers noted increased numbers of dead hares. One was obtained for post-mortem examination. It had no discharges from orifies and no diarrhoeic staining. Internally there was a notable absence of body fat (i.e. none around the kidneys or in the mesenteries, which were glass-clear). Parenchymal organs were normal in appearance and no abnormality was evident in the thoracic organs. Pale foci were seen throughout much of the small intestine, visible through the outer mesenteric surface (55a), and distinct pale patches were evident in the mucosa when the small bowel was opened (55b).

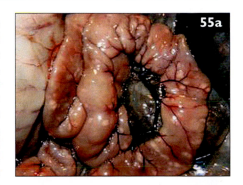

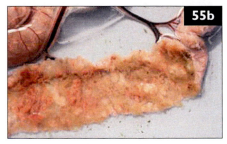

i. What are these pale foci in the small bowel?
ii. How commonly are they seen, and are they a cause of mortality?
iii. What test can be done to validate the diagnosis?

56 In a large-scale bird oiling incident (56), triage is necessary to ensure that as many birds with a high chance of recovery as possible are treated.

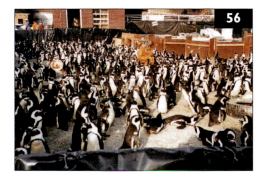

i. What is the first priority in treatment?
ii. When should birds be washed?
iii. What is the best way to clean oiled birds?
iv. What parameters need to be checked before release?

55 i. Massive clusters of mucosal coccidial oocysts (*Eimeria* spp.).
ii. Some degree of intestinal coccidiosis is present in most wild hares and they develop an immunity with time. Massive infestations are the commonest cause of death in young hares in their first autumn, particularly when environmental conditions are damp. The majority of the lesions are in the small intestine, with fewer in the large bowel, which is probably why diarrhoea is often not a feature.
iii. The laboratory examination of faeces will confirm high numbers of oocysts.

56 i. Stabilization (removal of excess oil, stabilization of body temperature, oral administration of an enteric coating agent, rehydration, nutritional support).
ii. Not until they have been stabilized (normal body temperature; weight within 10% of normal; normal hydration level, PCV, total proteins, blood glucose; absence of apparent infectious disease). If the oil will cause chemical burns (e.g. diesel, jet fuel) or birds are severely coated, a quick (maximum five minutes) wash should be given soon after admission.
iii. With detergent and hot water. The water should be at about 42°C in order to clean the bird quickly without scalding or cooling. The water must be fresh, not salt water, and not too hard. Washing should continue until the wash water remains clean. Once all the oil has been removed, the feathers must be rinsed until all the detergent is removed and water is beading on the feathers. The bird is then patted dry with towels and left in a dimly lit, quiet drying cage or drying room.
iv. Normal weight and body condition for the species, age, sex and time of year; an adequate PCV; a normal level of waterproofing. The release site must be checked (appropriate habitat for the species; free of oil; any necessary permissions in place to release the birds).

57 A hedgehog presented because it was dragging both hindlimbs (**57a**). Although the forelimbs were unaffected, it was unable to curl up when threatened and was only able to bristle and erect the spines of the cranial half of the body. The caudal body spines remained flat against the skin.

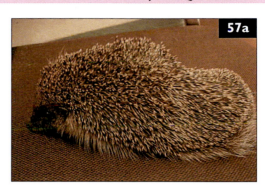

i. What is your diagnosis?
ii. How do the findings help to localize the lesion?
iii. How would you confirm the diagnosis?

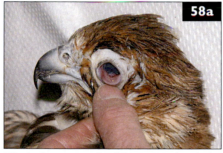
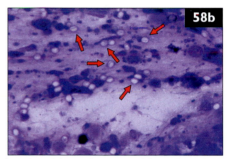

58 A three-month-old, captive bred, female saker falcon, kept in a falcon breeding facility, was presented with anorexia, respiratory difficulties and a bilateral ocular discharge (**58a**). The bird showed mild inspiratory and expiratory stridor and bilateral conjunctivitis. The bird was anaesthetized and the trachea was examined with an endoscope. A mild inflammation with mucus accumulation was observed in the trachea. Swabs were taken from the trachea and smears stained with a Diff-Quik® stain for cytology examination (**58b**).

i. What is your preliminary diagnosis in this bird based on the clinical signs and cytological findings?
ii. What diagnostic tests would be needed to confirm the aetiology?
iii. What are the route of infection and life cycle of the organism?

57 i. This hedgehog has spinal cord damage, most likely resulting from trauma, although other causes of spinal lesion, including inflammation, infection, neoplasia and intervertebral disc prolapse, are possible.

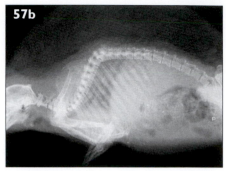

ii. The hindlimb paralysis with normal forelimb function is suggestive of a lesion caudal to the brachial outflow (or less likely a bilateral peripheral nerve problem). The location of the cut-off line between normal bristling spines and non-functional flattened spines indicates the level of the spinal cord damage, the underlying lesion being just cranial to this. This is equivalent to the panniculus reflex used to localize cord lesions in other species.

iii. Plain radiographs will usually reveal a spinal fracture or vertebral dislocation with cord transaction. In this case the radiograph shows fracture of the vertebral body T8, with associated compression on the vertebral canal causing denervation caudal to the lesion (57b).

58 i. Cryptosporidiosis caused by the coccidian parasite *Cryptosporidium* spp.. *C. baileyi*, *C. meleagridis* and *C. parvum* affect different avian species.

ii. The very small oocysts (4 × 8 µm) with sporozoites (arrows in 58b) can be found in cytology preparations of samples collected from air sacs, trachea or conjunctiva. Additional diagnostic methods include acid-fast staining, direct immunofluorescence staining, PCR or ELISA.

iii. The life cycle is direct and monoxenous (requires only one host). Oocysts containing four sporozoites are inhaled or ingested. Following release of the sporozoites, trophozoites are formed, as the epithelial cell encapsulates each sporozoite within its membrane. The trophozoite evolves to a meront type I, which releases 4–8 merozoites. At this point the merozoites can form new trophozoites, continuing the asexual cycle, or form a meront type II, which initiates the sexual phase of the cycle. The meront type II releases more merozoites and these become either microgamonts or macrogamonts. The microgamonts fertilize the macrogamonts, forming oocysts that may be excreted or reinfect the host. The endogenous phase occurs in the luminal border of epithelial cells of the respiratory, urinary and gastrointestinal tracts. Their location has been described as intracellular but extracytoplasmic. In the respiratory tract the parasite affects the mucociliary function, causing rhinitis, conjunctivitis, tracheitis, sneezing and dyspnoea.

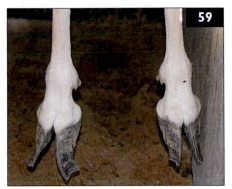

59 The feet of a scimitar-horned oryx are shown (59).
i. Describe the condition seen and the main causes of this problem.
ii. Name the types of common hoof problems that occur in captive wild ungulates.
iii. How would you deal with the problem in the individual animal and in the herd?

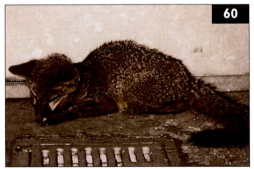

60 A grey fox suffering from classical rabies is shown (60). Appropriate virus–
animal interactions, including the host species' natural history, lead to major rabies
species reservoirs in various geographic regions. Briefly describe the major rabies
reservoir species for Southern Africa, Europe, Asia, North America and Latin and
South America.

59 i. Overgrown hooves. The causes are multifactorial and include genetics, enclosure size and substrate and nutrition. A combination of reduced exercise on poorly abrasive surfaces, wet autumn conditions and excess dietary protein are considered to contribute to the development of hoof problems in captive oryx. In their natural arid environment, free-living oryx range over large distances and abrasive surfaces. In comparison, captive oryx in zoos are kept in small grass enclosures. Even semi-free-living oryx in large reserves may not travel the same distances as wild animals, especially if they are provided with supplemental feeding.
ii. Overgrown hoofs, hoof cracks, cuticle overgrowth, solar abscess, contusions, penetrating wounds, laminitis, candidiasis and infectious pododermatitis.
iii. The individual animal needs appropriate repeated hoof trimming. Preventive measures within a herd include controlled breeding, enclosure design and adequate dietary management. In temperate climates the provision of larger, dry yard areas to overwinter stock may reduce the incidence of hoof pathology. Fine sand should be added to hard areas to act as an abrasive. Feeding stations could be moved around and enrichment techniques used to help stimulate movement.

60 Southern Africa. Since 1940 rabies virus has infected wildlife species via spillover from domestic dogs. Previously, viverrid species were the main reservoir. In some areas the jackal is the main reservoir, whereas in others it is the bat-eared fox and yellow mongoose. Endemic viverrid rabies viruses are also evolving over long periods amongst stable non-migratory populations.

Europe. Rabies is compartmentalized, with bats, red foxes and arctic foxes being the major reservoirs (the raccoon dog is also important). The red fox is the ideal rabies host, as flexible social structures and population dynamics promote high conspecific contact during relatively short periods of intensive intraspecific transmission. The serotine bat comprises more than 85% of bat rabies cases in Europe.

Asia. The major reservoir is the domestic dog, although foxes appear to be a major reservoir in the Middle East.

North America. Ninety per cent of cases occur in wildlife. Major North American/Canadian reservoirs are raccoons (the Atlantic and southeast), red fox (New England), arctic and red fox (Alaska), skunk, mainly striped (North Central, South Central and California, which are all distinct rabies variants), coyotes (Texas) and grey foxes (southwest).

The major reservoir in Latin and South America is the domestic dog, with the notable role of haematophagous bats (e.g. the vampire bat).

61 A post-weaning orphaned common or harbour seal is presented to your practice by members of a marine animal welfare association (61a). It is tachypnoeic, with harsh lung sounds. There is a mucoid nasal discharge and live worms approximately 5 cm long are noted in the faeces.

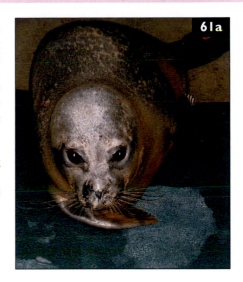

i. What is your diagnosis?
ii. How would you proceed in managing this case?
iii. What further diagnostic procedures might you carry out?

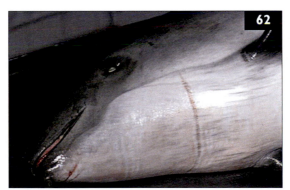

62 You are asked to carry out a gross post-mortem examination of a stranded cetacean and collect relevant samples. Closer examination of the carcase reveals a number of lesions that lead you to be suspicious of bycatch (i.e. entanglement in fishing nets) as the likely cause of death (62). Although most bycaught cetaceans do not strand alive, occasionally this may occur. What gross lesions may lead to you to such a conclusion?

61 i. The seal is hydrated, as evidenced by the tear marked circles around the eyes and, while underweight, it is not emaciated. It is in ventral recumbency, which at rest can be associated with some respiratory effort. The mucoid nasal discharge and faecal worms are strongly indicative of clinical lungworm infestation. *Parafilaroides gymnurus* and *Otostrongylus circumlitis* are seen in this species, with adult worms and larvae coughed up and swallowed, often found regurgitated or passed in faeces.

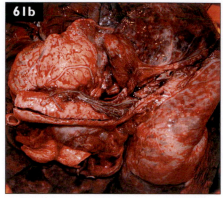

Secondary bacterial bronchopneumonia is likely and the presence of the worms will cause tissue destruction, haemorrhage, inflammation, mucus production and oedema (**61b**, *O. circumlitis* in the bronchial tree).

ii. Do not give anthelmintic drugs prior to stabilization. Rapid lungworm die off can cause local inflammation, anaphylaxis and simple blockage of the airways in heavily infested individuals. Any fluid deficits should be addressed and administration of NSAIDs or glucocorticoids, mucolytics, bronchodilators and appropriate broad-spectrum antibiotics commenced before giving moxidectin or ivermectin at standard doses.

iii. Chest radiography is of limited use due to the subcutaneous fat layer in older juveniles and the difficulty of achieving inspiratory views and good positioning without general anaesthesia. Microscopic analysis of faeces or sputum is useful in diagnosing less overt infestations or establishing whether animals have been successfully treated.

62 Lesions associated with bycatch tend to be skin wounds and deeper trauma associated with capture in multifilament and particularly monofilament netting. These include encircling skin abrasions on the beak/rostrum (see **62**), flippers and flukes, multiple evenly spaced parallel incisions in the skin and, possibly, cleanly cut-off fins or tail flukes. Other signs that are suspicious, but not specific, for bycatch include evidence of a recent meal, mandibular fractures (usually seen post mortem) and bruising in submandibular and periscapular subcutaneous tissues. Other signs that are more likely to be seen in dead strandings due to bycatch are lesions consistent with death by immersion, including epicardial petechial haemorrhages, froth in the bronchi and bullae in the lung parenchyma. Some of these lesions also may be seen as a consequence of live stranding.

63 A wildlife hospital reports that the blackbird fledglings they are hand rearing are making an abnormal gurgling or clicking respiratory noise. What is the most likely cause of the problem, and how would you investigate this further?

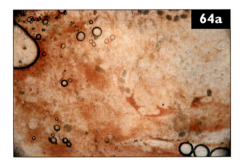

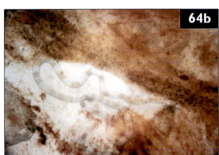

64 A hedgehog rehabilitator has over 40 hedgehogs, all admitted as 'out during the day and too small to hibernate: under 500g bodyweight' during the autumn. On admission they were given a proprietary pet store puppy and kitten dewormer at the package dose recommended for puppies and kittens, fed a mixture of dog and cat food, and were putting on weight satisfactorily,

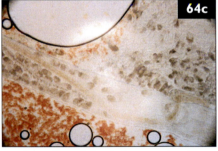

but in the last five days, eight hedgehogs have been found dead. Some animals are coughing or sneezing and some had shown a brief reduction in appetite before death. Three are presented for necropsy, but all are suffering from some degree of decomposition. On necropsy the abdominal contents are autolysed. However, it can be seen that there are areas of atelectasis and emphysema in the lungs. Smears made from the cut surface of the lungs are examined microscopically under low power (**64a–c**).
i. What can you see in these photos?
ii. What is your diagnosis, what treatment would you give, and what advice would you offer the rehabilitator?

63 Syngamiasis is a common parasitic infection of birds, particularly in juveniles of the *Corvidae* and *Turdidae* families. The condition is colloquially known as 'gapeworm' infection and is an important concern for game bird and intensive poultry management systems.

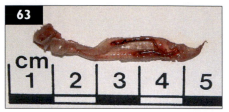

The blood-red coloured adult stage of the parasite, *Syngamus trachea*, is found in the trachea, partially obstructing the major airways (63). Infection may be asymptomatic or it can lead to clinical disease. Clinical signs include open mouth breathing, head shaking, abnormal respiratory noise and serious respiratory compromise in cases with heavy infection. Weight loss and anaemia may also occur. The parasite life cycle is indirect, with an invertebrate paratenic host (e.g. earthworm, snail or slug).

Standard parasitological faecal examination, using individual or pooled samples for group-housed birds, should be performed. Infection is diagnosed based on the characteristic bioperculate appearance of the ova (90 × 50 μm). General clinical examination, history taking, and other diagnostic screening procedures may be required to evaluate differential diagnoses for avian respiratory disease.

64 i. Adults and larvae of two species of lungworm. *Crenosoma striatum* is a live bearing worm and adults are found in the trachea, bronchi, bronchioles and alveolar ducts. The caudal part of an adult worm, containing embryonated eggs surrounded by newly hatched live larvae, can be seen in 64c. *Capillaria aerophila* is a smaller, thinner worm bearing bipolar eggs. Adults are often found in the epithelium of the bronchi, bronchioles and trachea. Both live larvae and bipolar eggs can be seen throughout the slides (64a, b).

ii. A heavy infestation of lungworms, which is the likely cause of death. Because of their low bodyweight, the recommended puppy and kitten dose of dewormer per unit of bodyweight will be low and ineffective. Using allometric scaling, several anthelmintics have been used successfully to treat lungworm in hedgehogs, including oral fenbendazole (100 mg/kg for 5 days), levamisole (27 mg/kg s/c 3 times at 48-hour intervals) and ivermectin (up to 3 mg/kg s/c). All these doses are considerably higher than those for domestic species.

The effectiveness of worming can be checked rapidly by examination of a faecal smear post treatment. Because shedding of eggs and larvae can be intermittent, it is better to examine several smears over a period of time.

65 Eight flamingos have just arrived at a zoo after a long journey. When they are let out of the burlap bags they have been transported in, they cannot stand up.
i. What is the likely problem?
ii. What is the treatment?
iii. What is the prognosis?
iv. How can this problem be prevented in the future?

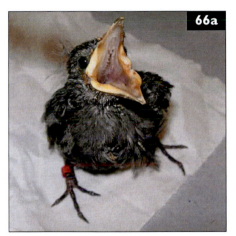
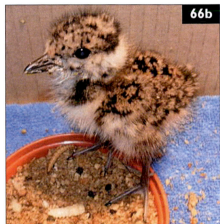

66 Fledgling birds are often found alone and apparently abandoned by their parents. Most should be left alone or moved into the safety of cover nearby and the parent will usually return. Many are mistakenly 'rescued' and taken into care for hand rearing. If presented with juvenile birds that cannot be returned to the wild or which are genuinely orphaned, it is important to try to identify the species. All birds can broadly be divided into altricial (66a) and precocial types as shown (66b).
i. What do these terms mean?
ii. How do these affect the way they are hand reared?
iii. Why must human contact be kept to a minimum, especially in precocial species?

65 i. 'Leg cramp', probably a form of capture myopathy. It is seen in long-legged birds of all sizes, including waders (shorebirds), which have had their legs kept in a flexed position for a prolonged period. This position reduces circulation; at the same time the bird may repeatedly try to straighten its legs, putting considerable stress on the muscles.

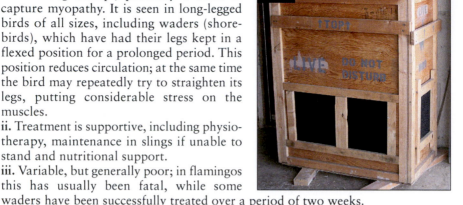

ii. Treatment is supportive, including physiotherapy, maintenance in slings if unable to stand and nutritional support.

iii. Variable, but generally poor; in flamingos this has usually been fatal, while some waders have been successfully treated over a period of two weeks.

iv. Long-legged birds should always be transported with their legs extended, preferably standing in individual crates of an appropriate size (**65**). If restrained for treatment, they should be held with their legs extended, keeping a finger between the legs at the hocks to stop damage from the legs rubbing against one another. The legs can be flexed for a short period if necessary, but should never be forced into a flexed position, and should be returned to an extended posture as soon as possible.

66 i. Altricial birds are hatched naked and blind and are totally dependent on the parents for food and warmth. Precocial birds are more developed when they hatch and are able to feed themselves soon afterwards, although they still rely on parents for warmth and protection.

ii. Altricial nestlings will usually gape (open their mouth) for food and must be hand fed regularly throughout the day with a high quality food placed directly into the beak. Precocial birds are able to feed themselves if suitable food is offered, although some initial encouragement may be required. Additionally, precocial birds are fully feathered and mobile, whereas altricial birds are featherless when they hatch and require more warmth and care. In general, the hand rearing of precocial birds is less labour intensive.

iii. Precocial juveniles follow their parents soon after hatching and have a relatively short time period in which to recognize and form an attachment to them. They are therefore prone to imprinting when artificially reared and can mistake the foster human for the parent bird, especially if newly hatched. This learned association, once formed, is irreversible and can lead to long-term behavioural problems.

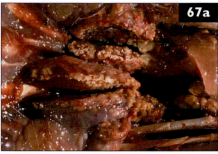

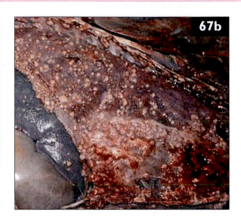

67 These images (67a, retropharyngeal lymph nodes; 67b, thoracic cavity) are from a 3.5-year-old female white-tailed deer shot in Michigan, USA.
i. Describe the lesions seen.
ii. Name the most likely causative organism. What is the aetiology of the disease in this species?

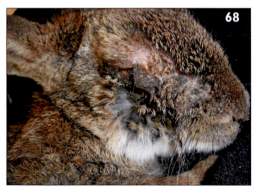

68   This wild rabbit (68) has been brought in to your veterinary surgery by a member of the public who is keen to try and treat it.
i. What is the most likely cause of this rabbit's condition?
ii. When was this disease first introduced into Europe, and why?
iii. How is it spread between rabbits?
iv. Would you advise treating this rabbit?

67 i. The retropharyngeal lymph nodes demonstrate discrete, multiple nodular lesions on their surfaces, infiltrating into the parenchyma and also affecting adjacent structures There are multiple, diffuse, discrete, focal, nodular lesions on the lung surface and thoracic cavity surfaces. A central, walled-off area of mineralization and caseous necrosis surrounded by a thick mononuclear

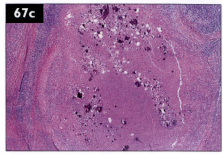

inflammatory infiltrate interspersed with areas of fibrosis is shown in the histological section 67c.

ii. Mycobacterial infection, which in white-tailed deer can be subacute to chronic. Lesions may be confined to the superficial lymph nodes of the head, such as the submandibular, the parotid and particularly the retropharyngeal lymph nodes, suggesting both oral and respiratory transmission pathways. *M. bovis* persists in tonsillar crypts and can be shed via nasal and oral secretions. In contrast to cattle, many infections in white-tailed deer have a tendency to abscess formation with purulent discharge, although granuloma formation is also seen. Infections increase with age and can range from no gross lesions visible to systemic involvement of multiple organs and tissues. The most common sites for lesions are the lymph nodes and associated structures of the head and the lung and thoracic wall.

68 i. Myxomatosis, caused by the myxoma pox virus.
ii. It was introduced to control wild rabbits in France in 1952, with subsequent spread to the British Isles. The virus's natural host is the South American forest rabbit.
iii. By arthropod vectors, mainly the rabbit flea (*Spilopsyllus cuniculi*) in the UK, but can also be mosquito borne. The flea's life cycle is linked to the reproductive status of the female rabbit. This leads to heavy flea infestation of the young and so they are particularly susceptible to infection with the virus. The virus does not replicate in the vector, but in the infection site, spreading to regional lymph nodes.
iv. The majority of rabbits die within two weeks due to secondary bacterial septicaemia. There are anecdotal reports of successful treatment with supportive care consisting of systemic antibiotics, fluid therapy and provision of warmth. However, captivity is highly stressful for a wild rabbit. Given that the prognosis is so poor, euthanasia is generally recommended.

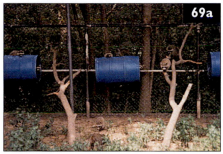

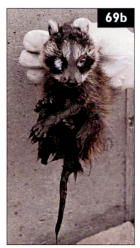

69 You are called to a wildlife rehabilitation centre that rehabilitates and rears several hundred raccoon kits each year. As soon as the kits are weaned (approximately 7–8 weeks of age), they are moved into large outdoor pens where they are group housed (69a). On the morning you are called, the rehabilitator discovered two dead raccoons in the cage and one that has oculonasal discharge and diarrhoea (69b).
i. What are your two main differential diagnoses?
ii. What in-house test(s) can be done to differentiate the two, and what clinical signs are seen with each?
iii. What definitive diagnostic tests can be done?

70 This seal pup was found on a beach off the east coast of Scotland with an obvious neck injury (70).
i. What species of seal is it?
ii. What may have caused the injury?
iii. How would you treat the lesion?

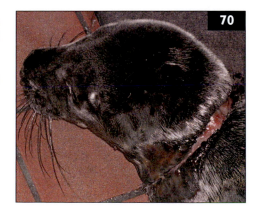

69 i. Canine distemper virus (CDV) and raccoon parvovirus (RPV). (Raccoons can also get feline parvovirus [FPV] and mink enterititis virus [MEV]), so these could be included in the differential list).

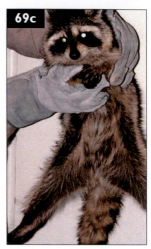

69c

ii. An in-house faecal ELISA test for canine parvovirus will often show a positive result for RPV, FPV or MEV, so a positive result can be used to rule out CDV. A negative result does not necessarily mean that a parvovirus is not present. Clinically, both CDV and the parvoviruses may exhibit oculonasal discharges and unkempt fur. Raccoons with CDV often exhibit central nervous system signs, including hyperreflective tapedae (**69c**) and ataxia, with varying degrees of other neurological signs including circling, 'chewing gum seizures' and full tonic–clonic seizures. Parvoviral infections usually manifest with gastrointestinal signs, including diarrhoea and distended, gas-filled bowel loops. Evidence of hypermotility (plications) in the small intestines is commonly seen on post-mortem examination.

iii. Virus isolation or histopathology on post-mortem tissues (urinary bladder preferred for CDV; small intestines preferred for parvovirus).

70 i. A common or harbour seal. The muzzle is short and the nostrils form a 'V' shape. This species is smaller and has a paler coat than grey seals, the other species seen frequently in the region.

ii. The injury encircles the neck and is most likely due to entanglement (e.g. in netting or fishing line).

iii. Perform a complete physical examination to assess for other pathology. Remove any material from around the neck and investigate the extent of the lesion. Wounds commonly become infected and may result in septicaemia. Deep wounds require surgical investigation and débridement. Systemic antibiotics are necessary if deep injuries or obvious infection are present (e.g. amoxicillin, 10 mg/kg p/o q12h [7 mg/kg i/m q24h]; amoxicillin–clavulanate, 12.5 mg/kg p/o q12h [8.75 mg/kg i/m q24h]). If a discharge is present or healing does not progress satisfactorily, take swabs for culture and sensitivity. Cleaning with saline and/or dilute antiseptic (e.g. chlorhexidine, povidone–iodine) on a daily basis will facilitate healing. If the rehabilitation centre has facilities, addition of salt to water in a shallow pool may be helpful. Provide analgesia (e.g. carprofen, 2 mg/kg p/o q12–24h) and other supportive care (e.g. assist feeding with liquidized fish) if necessary. This lesion did not require surgical débridement. Systemic antibiotics and topical antiseptics resulted in healing within five weeks.

71 You are called to the scene of a road accident involving an adult deer. What do you need to consider when preparing to capture and handle this animal (71)?

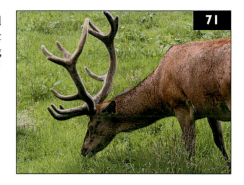

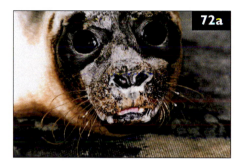

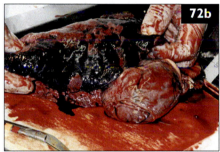

72 Two harbour seal pups are found on the beach on the same day (72a). They are considered to be weaned, independent pups of the current year by their size, and are in moderate to good body condition. Both are brought into care at a local wildlife centre. Both have respiratory distress and mucopurulent nasal and ocular discharge, and are dull and unresponsive. One has a dry crepitus

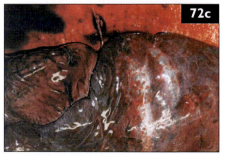

detectable on palpation of the neck and thorax. The animal with crepitus suffers convulsions and dies shortly after admission. You perform a necropsy, which reveals subcutaneous emphysema and the lesions shown (72b, c).
i. What lesions can you see on the gross necropsy?
ii. What is the likely diagnosis, and what would be your differential list?
iii. How would you confirm your diagnosis?
iv. What tissues other than those showing lesions would be useful for diagnosis?

71 Deer are potentially dangerous when handled and consideration must be made for the safety of those involved in handling casualties. Handling and capture must be well planned and involve suitable handling equipment, including sedative or anaesthetic drugs and darting equipment. Provision for euthanasia should be available, including the services of a marksman.

Equipment should include: thick blankets or rugs for covering the head of all species and restraint of smaller species; cargo or freight netting for restraint of larger species; ropes for hobbling larger species; crates or boxes for housing smaller species. Drugs may include: medetomidine or xylazine; etorphine; atipamazole; ketamine; diazepam; intravenous fluids (lactated Ringer's solution, glucose saline [for capture myopathy]); pentobarbitone or secobarbital plus cinchocaine (for euthanasia).

Consideration of the necessity of handling and the extent to which the deer is handled must be made. Most deer, unless trapped in some way or severely injured, will have vacated the site of an accident long before a veterinarian arrives. Injured deer must be carefully triaged, ideally from a distance or following sedation. Deer are poor patients in captivity, being less easy to handle and more susceptible to stress and capture myopathy than other species. If immediate release is not possible, then euthanasia is often preferable to capture, transportation, treatment and rehabilitation.

72 i. Severe consolidation combined with emphysema.
ii. Phocine distemper (PD). The combination of clinical signs of subcutaneous emphysema and convulsions, and the gross necropsy findings are typical of PD. Canine distemper (CD) can affect seals, and epizootics of Baikal and Caspian seals have been attributed to CD, with similar clinical and pathological findings. Phocine herpesvirus has been responsible for outbreaks of disease in seals in rehabilitation and has produced a range of neurological and respiratory clinical signs not dissimilar to PD and similar lesions on gross necropsy. Verminous pneumonia and associated secondary bacterial infections can produce severe respiratory distress and subcutaneous emphysema, and variable oculonasal discharge.
iii. Virus isolation and PCR can confirm the diagnosis. In the acute stages of the disease, animals may not have seroconverted. Morbilliviruses induce immuno-suppression and parasite loads can be high in affected animals, so care must be taken to identify the primary cause of disease. Histology should reveal typical morbillivirus inclusions.
iv. Like CDV, the bladder wall is a target tissue for virus replication and is often rich in inclusion bodies, so is a useful sample to take for histology.

73 Phocine distemper, caused by phocine distemper virus (PDV) is diagnosed in two harbour seal pups brought into a wildlife rescue centre in the UK.
i. What are the implications for wild seals, other seals in the wildlife centre and other animals?
ii. Is this disease potentially zoonotic?

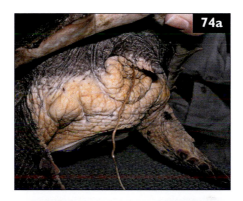

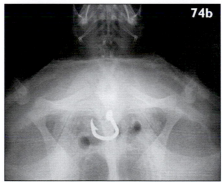

74 A loggerhead sea turtle strands with a fishing line evident on clinical examination protruding from the cloaca (**74a**). On radiographic examination a hook is seen in the distal part of the oesophagus (**74b**).
i. What is the prognosis in this case?
ii. What treatment is indicated?

73 i. Phocine distemper has occurred as an epizootic outbreak twice in the eastern Atlantic, the Baltic and North Sea regions, in 1988 and again in 2002. In 1988 there was a mortality of up to 50% of populations of harbour seals in the Wash and the coast of Holland (North Sea). In the 2002 outbreak mortality was lower, at around 18%. Grey seals were little affected and appear to have a high degree of innate resistance to infection with PDV. On the eastern seaboard of the USA (the western Atlantic) an unusual mortality event (UME) in seals was declared in 2006/2007, believed to be associated with morbillivirus infection. The mortality associated with this event was not in the proportions seen in the eastern Atlantic, although interestingly, a number of grey seals have been affected.

ii. PDV is spread by aerosol and is highly infectious. CDV can infect seals and a range of other carnivores, but there is no evidence of field infection of other carnivores with PDV. However, precautions should be put in place, particularly to exclude dogs from contact with potentially affected seals, both within rehabilitation centres and on the shoreline where affected wild seals may strand. PDV has shown no potential as a zoonosis.

74 i. Extremely poor, especially because the hook is embedded in the oesophagus and the attached fishing line has already been ingested through the intestinal tract. The peristaltic movements of the intestines pull the line gradually, tensing up the animal's gastrointestinal tract as a concertina effect. The line causes haemorrhage and necrosis of the stomach and intestines, and eventually results in perforations, peritonitis and subsequent death.

ii. Immediate emergency treatment involves cutting the line from the hook and performing a coeliotomy, surgically accessing different parts of the gastrointestinal tract in order to cut the line at different levels and so prevent it cutting through the walls of the intestine. If the turtle is not strong enough to survive such a surgical procedure, the coeliotomy should not be carried out. In this case the line is left to transit through the intestines, causing further necrosis and haemorrhage. The animal may eventually recover from these lesions in the intestines and stomach; however, until it does it will show symptoms of severe malabsorptive protein-losing enteropathy. Supportive care and nursing are essential during this period.

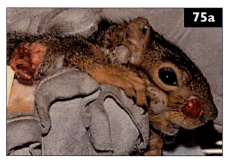

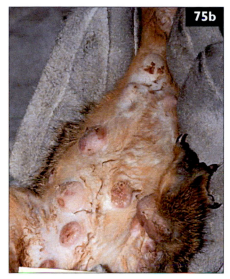

75 This female, juvenile fox squirrel is found with raised lesions over a large portion of the body (75a, b). Many of the lesions are open, and while the animal does occasionally scratch at an open lesion, it does not appear overly pruritic. The animal is eating normally and has no gross evidence of ecto-parasites.

i. What is the cause of the dermal lesions on this fox squirrel?
ii. How is this condition transmitted, and what species may be affected?
iii. What is the recommended treatment?

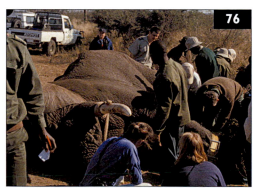

76 A wild elephant is anaesthetised prior to translocation (76). An international study found that that 25% of translocated wildlife species were not given a physical examination by a veterinarian or biologist before moving. How would you draw up a translocation plan for a group of animals?

75   i. Fibromatosis, also known as squirrel pox, which is caused by the squirrel fibroma virus, a poxvirus closely related to the myxoma and Shope's fibroma viruses that infect rabbits. A skin biopsy from an affected squirrel demonstrates the intracytoplasmic inclusion body typical of most pox viruses (75c).

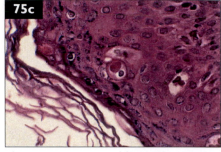

ii. Mosquitoes are known to transmit this disease between squirrels. As with other pox viruses, additional routes of transmission could include direct animal-to-animal passage (through direct contact with open lesions) and/or ectoparasites such as fleas, lice and mites. Fox squirrels, eastern and western grey squirrels and woodchucks are naturally infected; domestic rabbits have been experimentally infected.

iii. Treatment consists largely of supportive care. Open lesions may be cleaned and anecdotal evidence suggests that the application of topical iodine will help prevent secondary infections, dry the lesions and reduce the healing time.

76 (1) Prepare a detailed description of the wild animal translocation to be assessed. This should include objective signalment of animals shipped, timing of the translocation, source and destination ecosystems and differences between the two, capture/handling/medical protocols to be employed and a summary of the health, economic and ecological risks involved. (2) Identify the potential health hazards associated with the proposed animal translocation. This should include analyses of all diseases the animals are exposed and susceptible to at the point of origin and destination and their effects on other species. Also include disease risks in transit and any vaccinations and other biological preparations the animals have been exposed to. Include non-infectious hazards (nutritional, toxicological, conflict with human activities) at the destination. (3) Make an assessment of each health hazard identified. (4) Make an overall statement of the risk involved in the translocation. (5) Make a statement about any additional risks involved not specifically covered when identifying potential health hazards (e.g. damage to the environment, change in the nature or type of biomass available for cover from predators due to increased grazing pressure). (6) Make recommendations to reduce the risks.

77 A bald eagle nestling being sampled by biologists in the USA as part of an ecotoxicological study examining persistent organic pollutants in tertiary avian predators is shown (77).

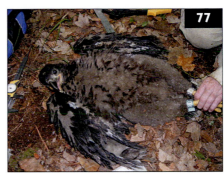

i. What effects are caused by polychlorinated biphenyls (PCBs) in avian species, and what is the mechanism of action?

ii. What might be some of the issues associated with proving negative impacts on reproduction in these species?

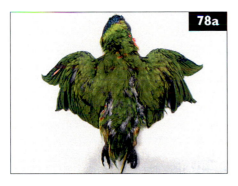

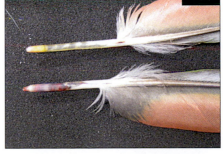

78 A wild rainbow lorikeet was brought to a wildlife rehabilitation hospital in Queensland, Australia.

i. Describe the clinical signs (78a–c), and provide a likely aetiology.

ii. What is the significance of the disease in this particular species?

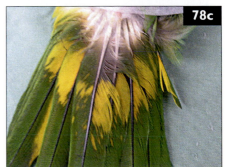

77 i. PCBs are mixtures of 209 commercial congeners released from chemical and combustion processes. They have been related to decreased reproductive success in wild mammals, birds and fish. The mechanism of action is incompletely understood. Coplanar PCBs operate through the aryl hydrocarbon receptor as antioestrogens. The antioestrogenic effects may be related to decreased oestrogen receptor number rather than to direct binding of PCBs to the oestrogen receptor. PCBs may also act by altering gene expression of the oestrogen receptor. Another mode of action may be to alter enzyme induction. PCBs also disrupt thyroid and adrenal gland homeostasis, which may play a role in reproductive toxicity. Some PCB congeners have conformational properties similar to DDT and are weakly oestrogenic. Therefore, multiple mechanisms of action are occurring.

ii. The evidence for PCB reproductive toxicity in avian species relies on correlation of field observations of reproductive success with residue analysis of tissues and eggs of exposed birds. PCBs have been associated with abnormal breeding behaviour of gulls. Isolating a cause and effect with wildlife is difficult, as many mixtures of chemicals can cause similar effects. Another difficulty is the lack of uniformity with the way study data is presented and the time frame over which long-term effects can be assessed.

78 i. There is loss of tail and distal primary flight feathers and abnormal feather growth. The plucked feathers show typical structural changes of a pinched calamus/rachis and necrosis. Feather colour has changed in areas from green to pale yellow, especially on the tail. These signs are consistent with psittacine beak and feather disease (PBFD) caused by a circovirus

ii. Rainbow lorikeets and scaly-breasted lorikeets are by far the most common wild birds in southeast Queensland that are presented with PBFD. Affected birds are typically young (determined by a dark beak colour). Research suggests that lories carry a variant form of the virus (named psittacine circovirus 2, Ps-CV 2). Nucleic acid sequence analysis confirmed that the virus in lories has sufficient nucleic acid differences that it is not detected using proprietary nucleic acid primers to the original documented virus (now known as psittacine circovirus 1, Ps-CV 1). As there are reports of lorikeets surviving documented disease, it is thought that this variant may be less pathogenic than disease caused by Ps-CV 1.

79 i. What are the two most common ectoparasites found in juvenile tawny owls (in the UK).

ii. What is the significance of such parasites?

iii. What is unusual about the parasitism shown (**79a**), and how should such cases be treated?

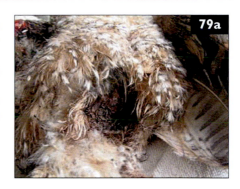

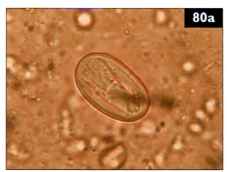

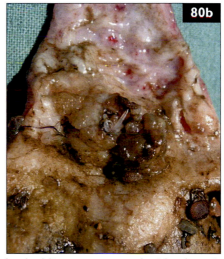

80 A group of eight-week-old shelducks on a freshwater pool during a hot summer became increasingly dull, lethargic and inappetent. A pooled faecal sample examined by direct microscopy revealed oval thick-walled helminth eggs measuring approximately 50 × 30 µm (**80a**). All the ducklings were treated with a broad-spectrum anthelmintic, but failed to improve. Post-mortem examination revealed thickening at the junction between the proventriculus and the gizzard (isthmus) with excess mucus production (**80b**). Worms were present in these lesions in some of the birds.

i. What are these nematodes?

ii. What was the significance of the hot weather?

iii. Why was anthelmintic treatment ineffective in these birds?

iv. What management factors could be used to reduce disease in subsequent years?

79 i. Lice and hippoboscids. The parasite load increases during the breeding season when an increase in stressors coincides with a build-up of parasites in the nest.

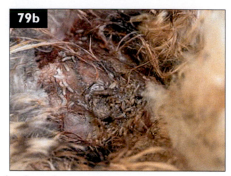

ii. Avian lice (order *Mallophaga*) feed mostly on feather debris. A build-up of feather lice is commonly seen in debilitated birds; healthy birds can reduce lice burdens by regular preening. Irritation and restlessness may be seen, progressing to loss of condition and feather damage in more severe cases. Hippoboscids (flat flies) are dorsoventrally flattened to facilitate movement through the bird's plumage. They cause pruritis, suck blood and transmit *Haemoproteus* and trypanosomes, as well as some parasitic mites. Heavy parasite loads can result in anaemia.

iii. The young tawny owl is suffering from fly strike (myiasis), which is relatively uncommon in birds, but may be seen in association with open wounds or soiled plumage and skin. Dirty nests may attract flies and chicks may present with myiasis. Affected birds are often severely debilitated and in shock. Where this is the case (as in **79b**, where second- and third-stage larvae are seen in an ulcerated abdominal wound with extensive tissue damage), euthanasia is recommended. Early cases will usually only have eggs or first-stage larvae present, and should undergo thorough wound debridement under general anaesthesia, removing all maggots. Use of permethrin products may also be indicated.

80 i. *Echinuria (Acuaria) uncinata*, which commonly affects juvenile waterfowl.
ii. The intermediate host for this parasite is primarily the water flea (*Daphnia* spp.), which rapidly reproduces in hot weather, increasing the potential for disease spread to waterfowl.
iii. The nematodes cause fibrous nodular thickening of the isthmus, which is often irreversible and permanently impairs digestion. Therefore, treatment with an anthelmintic when this scarring is already present will have little beneficial effect.
iv. Management factors are primarily aimed at reducing the number of intermediate hosts. Reproduction of the water fleas can be reduced by increasing the flow rate of the water or completely draining and refilling the pools with freshwater. Regular routine anthelmintic treatment of waterfowl, especially during the summer months, may help reduce any damage caused by the worms.

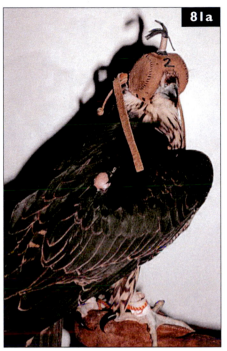

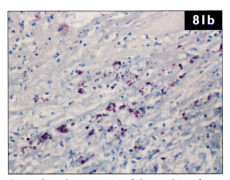

81 A female peregrine falcon (**81a**) from a rehabilitation centre was presented. Clinical examination revealed weight loss, inappetence, a change in faecal consistency, poor pectoral muscle condition and the presence of palpable subcutaneous nodules in the neck/crop region. Candidiasis was confirmed from a saline crop swab examined microscopically. A biopsy from a subcutaneous nodule in the neck was put in formalin and submitted for histology (Ziehl–Neelsen stain; **81b**). Haematology results showed a moderate leucocytosis with marked heterophilia and moderate monocytosis.

i. What lesion can be seen in the falcon?

ii. What is your provisional diagnosis, and what other test(s) would you recommend to confirm the diagnosis in this bird?

iii. What are the causative agent (s) of this condition?

iv. What is the route of infection?

v. What are the differential diagnoses for progressive weight loss in a raptor?

vi. What are the implications for the rehabilitation centre?

82 You are the owner of a veterinary practice dealing with wildlife casualties on a regular basis. What would your considerations be in devising a health and safety policy for your staff for when dealing with wildlife casualties?

81 i. Carpal bursitis.

ii. Mycobacteriosis. The presence of small, acid-fast, rod-shaped bacteria in the histology section supports the diagnosis. Endoscopy and biopsy of internal granulomas is helpful. Cultures should be incubated at 37°C for 6–8 weeks. PCR has been used to identify *M. avium* complex mycobacteria in formalin-fixed and unfixed tissues.

iii. Several mycobacterial species can cause this disease in birds, principally *M. avium*, *M. intracellulare* and *M. genavense*. As *M. avium* and *M. intracellulare* share some common antigens, these species are often grouped and termed as *M. avium-intracellulare* complex. Other mycobacterial species belonging to the *M. tuberculosis* complex, including *M. tuberculosis* and *M. bovis*, may also cause lesions in birds. *M. avium* is the most commonly isolated mycobacterial species in raptors. *M. avium paratuberculosis* has been isolated from falcons in the Middle East following feeding with contaminated mutton.

iv. The usual route of infection is oral, via direct contact or contact with food or water contaminated with faeces of infected birds.

v. Includes aspergillosis and chlamydophilosis. These two diseases and candidiasis are often diagnosed concurrently.

vi. In view of the zoonotic potential, affected birds should be euthanased. In-contact birds should be investigated and quarantined. The bacteria remain infectious in the environment for many months, so thorough decontamination should be carried out.

82 Within the practice it will be necessary for certain groups of staff to carry out differing tasks involving wildlife casualties. These tasks should be specified and limited to each group. Staff performing a certain task should be trained and certified in that task. There should be a health and safety risk assessment for each task or group of tasks, including the procedure(s) to be carried out, the perceived risks (e.g. bites, scratches, kicks, infections) and the methods in place to prevent these risks. Protection against risks will undoubtedly include the provision of suitable protective clothing (e.g. gloves, aprons, masks, leather gauntlets) and handling equipment (e.g. crush cages, cat catchers). There should be consideration of the wildlife species that are both commonly and rarely seen and specific assessments relating to these should be drawn up. Diseases carried by the species treated, especially zoonotic infections, must be considered in the risk assessment, in particular with respect to choice of protective equipment and the disinfectants used. The need for prophylactic protection against serious infections (e.g. rabies vaccinations) should also be reviewed on a regular basis and made a requirement of handling certain species if such a risk is perceived.

83 An unconscious loggerhead sea turtle is brought to a marine animal rehabilitation centre by a trawl fisherman. On clinical examination you find that the animal is not moving, is reported to have not taken a breath for one hour and has no corneal, palpebral or cloacal reflexes and no pain response.

i. What is the prognosis in this case?

ii. Describe any appropriate emergency treatment and first aid procedures.

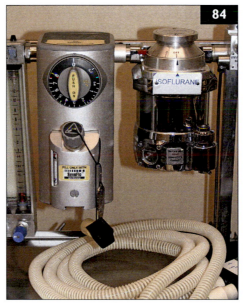

84 i. What are the similarities and differences between the gaseous agents in the vaporizer on the left of the picture (sevoflurane) and that on the right (isoflurane) (84)?

ii. What properties make these agents beneficial in the treatment of wildlife casualties?

83 i. Collapsed turtles can withstand long periods without breathing, and their heart rate can reduce to 1–2 beats/minute. A Doppler ultrasonic probe can be used to detect arterial blood flow on either side of the neck, but this may prove difficult. Unless the animal is showing signs of rigor mortis, it can be assumed it is still alive. The prognosis is guarded and depends on the response to emergency treatment.

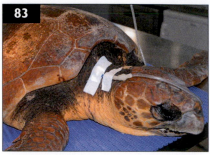

ii. Oxygen via an endotracheal tube and intravenous fluids and shock doses of steroids via the dorsal cervical sinus (83). The turtle should be warmed gradually to achieve a cloacal temperature of >20°C. It should be kept out of water, but moist at all times. With the turtle on its plastron, the caudal body is elevated to facilitate drainage of water from the lungs. Cardiopulmonary resuscitation is achieved by folding the animal's front flippers on either side of its neck and pushing the humerus–radius–ulnar joint into the body with the thumbs quickly and firmly, then letting go. This is repeated 4–5 times in quick succession to massage the heart. The fore-flippers are then extended cranially and then laterally on either side of the animal's body to encourage movement of air through the respiratory system. The whole cycle is then repeated. A drowned turtle may take several hours before it starts breathing voluntarily.

84 i. Both are fluorinated ethers. Both agents have low solubility, resulting in rapid anaesthetic induction, changes in depth of anaesthesia and recovery time. Sevoflurane, being the more soluble, has the most rapid effects. Isoflurane is a very potent anaesthetic (minimal alveolar concentration [MAC] 1.28% in the dog), allowing anaesthesia to be induced and maintained at relatively low concentrations. Sevoflurane is slightly less potent (MAC 2.1–2.4% in the dog), meaning that higher concentrations are needed. Both agents can be used for mask or chamber induction of anaesthesia. Isoflurane has a fairly strong, pungent odour that can result in breath holding and anxiety. Sevoflurane has a non-pungent and non-irritating odour, making it better tolerated. Anaesthesia with both isoflurane and sevoflurane results in less myocardial suppression than other agents (methoxyflurane, halothane). Both anaesthetic agents are primarily exhaled, with only 0.2% of isoflurane and 3% of sevoflurane being metabolized, making both agents an excellent choice for patients with renal or hepatic dysfunction.
ii. Their low solubility and rapid anaesthetic effects. Both agents have high safety profiles, making them useful in situations where the health status of the casualty is unknown. Sevoflurane is the most suitable agent for mask or chamber induction.

85   A red fox is found in a debilitated condition and dies shortly after being taken into care. You start a post-mortem examination and observe that areas of the lungs appear congested and consolidated, but there is also unusual yellowish brown discolouration (85a).
i. What is the likely cause of the observed changes?
ii. What would be the next stage in your post-mortem procedure?
iii. How would you investigate the lung lesions?
iv. What is the significance of this diagnosis in relation to the health of domestic animals?

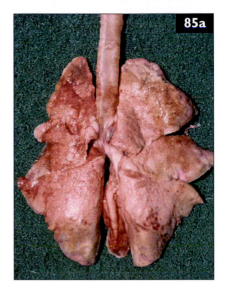

86   A hedgehog is presented with severe loss of spines (86). It is not pruritic. The skin is inflamed around the skirt, with a small amount of dried exudate and some crusts at the base of spines that can be plucked out easily. A light dusting of ectoparasites, just visible to the naked eye, is noted on the face.
i. What is the most likely diagnosis for this condition?
ii. How would you advise confirming this diagnosis and treating it?

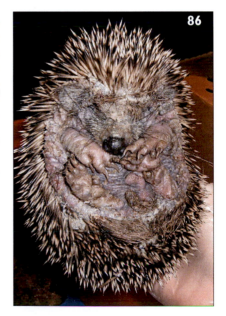

85 **i.** Infection with the heartworm *Angiostrongylus vasorum*.

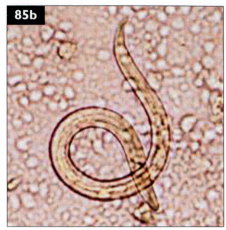

ii. Open the right ventricle and the pulmonary artery and look for adult nematodes (85a).

iii. Adult nematodes are not found on gross examination in every case, but evidence of infection can normally be proved by histopathological examination of lung. This will show the nematode eggs and first-stage larvae developing in the parenchyma. Another simple test is to make a scrape from the tracheal mucosa, place it on a microscope slide and examine with a low-power objective. This will often show first-stage larvae with their characteristic notched tail wriggling in the mucus (85b).

iv. *A. vasorum* is carried by foxes, often subclinically, and they are a reservoir of infection for domestic dogs. Slugs act as the principal intermediate host for the parasite and become infected by feeding on dog or fox faeces.

86 **i.** The ectoparasites are probably *Caparinia tripilis* mites, which can be vectors for the transmission of dermatophytosis. The clinical appearance (crusting skin and spine apex lesions, with spines being easily epilated on gentle traction) is typical of ringworm.

ii. Samples should be taken for microscopy and fungal culture. Multiple spines, or a brushing or scraping of the crusting lesions, or both, should be submitted for dermatophyte culture or performed in-house using standard dermatophyte test kits. Antibiosis may be required if, as in this case, there is significant secondary or coincidental bacterial dermatitis. Topical applications of natamycin or enilconazole, after pre-washing with povidone–iodine or chlorhexidine and miconazole shampoo, appear to be effective, but are highly labour intensive, requiring regular repeat washings. There is a moderate risk of human infection during this process. Oral administration of systemic antifungal agents (e.g. itraconazole or terbinafine) appears to be effective as long as reinfection from fomites and other infected animals can be prevented. An initial topical treatment and regular disinfection of the environment is advised. The *Caparinia* mites may be treated with fipronil or diluted ivermectin applied topically.

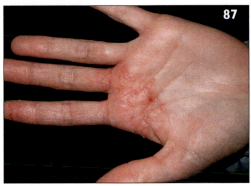

87   A client has a moderately severe dermatitis on one hand (87), which has developed since she started caring for the hedgehog in 86 one month ago. The lesions have worsened despite treatment with topical steroid cream. What advice would you give regarding this condition?

88   Several oriental white-backed vultures, found weak and collapsed in a roost adjacent to a cattle carcase dump in India, are rescued by a wildlife charity (88). All except one respond, over three days, to intravenous and subcutaneous fluids (0.9% saline) given at 2% bodyweight per day. A post-mortem examination performed on the dead bird found it to be in good condition with food in its gastrointestinal tract. Uric acid tophi were identified in several organs, giving an interim diagnosis of visceral gout and renal failure.

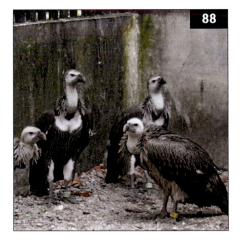

i. What may have caused the illness and death of the vultures?
ii. How could this be confirmed?
iii. What is the prognosis for the survivors?
iv. What would your recommendation be to the charity for subsequent management of the survivors?

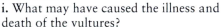

87 Dermatophytosis from hedgehogs is zoonotic and relatively easily transmitted if handling infected hedgehogs. Infection is introduced via spine microtrauma to the human skin. Latex gloves are not protective against this, and hedgehogs should be handled using thick gloves or a combination of latex gloves and impervious materials. The pattern of human infection is typically a small area of skin on the palms of the hands, spreading if untreated. Spread is increasingly rapid if a misdiagnosis as allergic dermatitis results in topical steroid application. Involvement of nail beds is possible, and the infection may be spread to other parts of the body via the infected skin of the hands. Typical ring-shaped lesions are not usually seen in this form, although they may be seen via contact with fomites. The client should be advised to see her GP as soon as possible, and given copies of any fungal testing results from infected animals.

88 i. They have probably eaten from an animal carcass treated with the NSAID diclofenac. Until recently this was freely available as a licensed veterinary product for use in ruminants. Its toxicity to scavenging vultures has led to a >99% decline in numbers of the *Gyps* species in the Indian subcontinent in the last decade.
ii. By analysis of tissue samples from the dead bird, in particular the liver, for diclofenac.
iii. Good. Birds that survive the initial effects on the renal system, which in part is dose-related, tend to show no permanent effects.
iv. Veterinary diclofenac products have been banned in a number of countries within the range of Asiatic *Gyps* species. Meloxicam is an alternative, having been demonstrated as safe for vultures and used therapeutically in several *Gyps* species. However, despite legal restrictions and extensive public information programmes, veterinary diclofenac use still persists (old or illegally imported stock and use of the human injectable form). Vultures are legally protected in India. One option would be to gain State Government permission to relocate survivors to a captive-breeding centre. These now hold over 200 birds, representing the three *Gyps* species native to India, with the aim of building up a captive population for release once diclofenac has been eliminated from the environment.

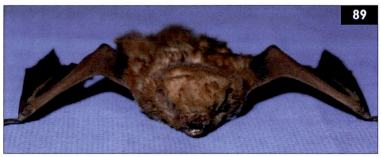

89 A client woke up to find this animal (89) in his bedroom.
i. What is this animal?
ii. What initial advice would you give to your client?

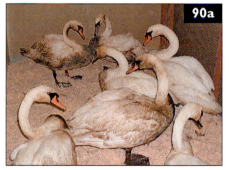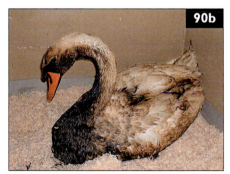

90 Seven mute swans (90a) are admitted to a local wildlife rehabilitation facility from the same body of water, a docks marina. They are preferring to spend time out of the water. On examination they are found to be a little underweight, with plantar thickening, and they have varying amounts of adherent dark oily material (90b).
i. What could this material be?
ii. Would you consider any diagnostic procedures in these cases?
iii. How would you manage these cases, both in initial treatment and before and after release?

89 i. A red bat.

ii. The bat should be captured safely and rabies testing of the bat arranged. One technique for capture involves closing all windows and doors, turning on the lights, and waiting for the bat to land. Wearing gloves (heavy, preferably thick leather), the bat should be covered with a coffee can or similar lidded container. A piece of cardboard is then slid underneath and the can turned right side up and sealed. If the bat is dead, it should be placed in double-layered plastic bags for submission to a diagnostic laboratory.

Anyone who has been in a room with a bat and is unsure whether an exposure took place should be considered exposed to rabies and should submit the bat for rabies testing. If the bat is not available, post-exposure rabies prophylaxis should be given. Most of the recent human rabies cases in the USA and Europe have been caused by bat variants of rabies virus (bat lyssaviruses), probably due to transmission via minor or unrecognized bat bites. Molecular epidemiological studies have linked most of these cases to lyssaviruses associated with insectivorous bats. In particular, virus variants associated with two relatively reclusive species, the silver-haired bat and the eastern pipistrelle, are the unexpected culprits of most cryptic cases of human rabies.

90 i. Mute swans permanently resident on inland watercourses or docks are often presented with plumage contamination from vegetable oil (discarded by food vendors), diesel or heavier engine oils. This appears to be engine oil.

ii. In general, mute swans seem to tolerate oiling better than seabirds, but diesel and heavier oils are potentially hepatotoxic and capable of causing haemolysis. Haematological and biochemical analysis may be worthwhile, especially in birds that do not recover well from the washing process.

iii. The swans should be housed indoors without access to water, as their waterproofing and thermal insulation are adversely affected by the oil. They should be given nutritional support and washed as soon as their general condition is satisfactory for release. Any significant foot lesions should be treated, and in cases where one foot is notably more affected than the other, weight bearing and function of the contralateral limb should be evaluated by examination and radiography. Thickened areas of the plantar hindlimb are common in swans on artificial substrates. Release of the birds to an alternative location is not likely to be helpful, as most will return to their original site. Ringing of the birds by appropriately trained personnel is advised to monitor their long-term health.

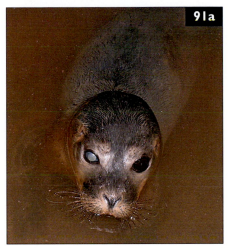

91   You are called to see a six-month-old common seal at a local wildlife rehabilitation centre. It is housed with one other seal in a semi-water-filled cubicle. Its left eye is almost completely closed and it is reluctant to eat. On examination under local anaesthesia in a darkened environment, you discover a central fluorescein-positive lesion, approximately 8 mm diameter, which has not extended as deep as Descemet's membrane, and a periphery of corneal oedema covering all the visible cornea (**91a**).
i. What is your diagnosis?
ii. What factors do you think could have played a part in its development?
iii. How would you treat this case, and what would have been the likely progression without treatment?
iv. What is the prognosis for release and post-release survival in this case?

92   Bait containing cyanide poison is placed in bait stations and bait bags in New Zealand. Warning notices are put up informing people when the bait stations and bags have been filled with bait and warning people not to handle the bait, to keep children under supervision at all times, not to allow dogs in to areas where bait has been placed and not to take any animals for eating. Which species is being targeted with the poisoned bait, and why?

91 i. Corneal oedema, which is common and marked in seals with corneal ulceration or damage.

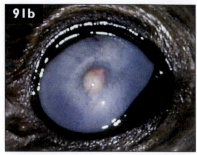

ii. Trauma (infighting with conspecifics, foreign material, handling of uncooperative individuals), primary or secondary bacterial infection.

iii. Rapid aggressive treatment with systemic NSAIDs and topical antibiosis is necessary to avoid permanent damage. Severe cases may benefit from fortified solutions of cephalosporins and/or gentamycin, made using ocular lubricant solutions. Systemic antibiotics may be required. Topical serum from the individual can assist healing. The animal should be kept in saline to keep the eyes moist. Repeated removal from water, for long enough for drops to stay in an adequate length of time, is stressful and impractical. Regular spraying of the eyes with saline via a plant mister may help. Conjunctival pedicle grafts may be placed to protect the cornea. Third eyelid flaps are less useful, but technically easier and more robust in a semi-aquatic environment postoperatively. Corneal rupture is a common sequela if the condition is left untreated.

iv. Corneal rupture and panophthalmitis in a grey seal is shown (**91b**). If this occurs, the prognosis for continued sight in that eye is grim. Although enucleation may be performed, the survival rates of visually challenged seals post release is unknown.

92 The brush-tailed possum, which was introduced into NZ in 1837 from Australia in order to establish fur farms. Some animals escaped from the farms and the species became well established. Possums are an important cause of damage to native vegetation. They consume bird eggs and chicks, thus contributing to the demise of native ground-nesting birds. Additionally, possums have become NZ's most significant wildlife reservoir for *Mycobacterium bovis* infection in cattle and deer. They are highly susceptible to *M. bovis* and although mostly solitary animals, they do share dens and have some social contact, allowing for spread of infection. Organisms are excreted via various routes, with respiratory spread and pseudo-vertical transmission from mother to offspring being considered the most important methods of transfer.

There has been large-scale possum eradication mostly through the use of poisoned bait. In some areas, culling has resulted in dispersal of infected possums and the creation of edge habitats with high levels of tuberculosis. Additional strategies, such as oral vaccination of possums, improved testing of livestock and consideration of other vector and reservoir species, have therefore been adopted.

93 Surveillance surveys in some areas of the USA have found the prevalence of *Mycobacterium bovis* in the wild white-tailed deer herd to be around 4–5%.
i. In what other wildlife species has this infection been diagnosed in this area, and what is the significance of this?
ii. List some other wild animal species that this infection has been diagnosed in worldwide.

94 List the criteria that should be met prior to the release of rehabilitated seal pups in order to ensure a successful outcome.

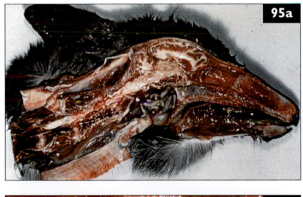

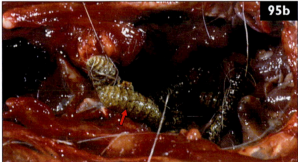

95 This parasite (95a, b, arrow) is commonly found in the nasopharynx of white-tailed deer in many locations throughout the USA. Name the genus, describe its life cycle, and comment on any pathogenic effects it may have on the host.

93 i. Infections have been diagnosed in various scavenging carnivore species (coyotes, red fox, raccoon, black bear) in the same area, but these are thought to be dead-end hosts not involved in persistence of the disease. *M. bovis* infections in cattle and other species often persist due to the presence of a wildlife reservoir. *M. bovis* infection in white-tailed deer in Michigan is an exception, but is strongly associated with long-term cultural attitudes to deer hunting and management in the region. These include management activities such as baiting, feeding and maintenance of focal high deer densities on large tracts of private land.

ii. *M. bovis* infections have been found in an enormous number of wild species worldwide, and include elk and white-tailed deer in Canada, bison in Canada, African buffalo in Kruger National Park, South Africa, feral Australian brushtail possums in New Zealand, feral ferrets in New Zealand, European badgers in the UK and Ireland, wild hoofstock in Spain and wild ungulates in Tanzania.

94
- Pups should be in good body condition and clinically well.
- Pups should be self-feeding on whole fish.
- Release should take place at the average expected weight at weaning. For grey seal pups this is 40–45 kg and for common seal pups it is 30–35 kg.

95 These nasopharyngeal bots are life stages of flies in the genus *Cephenymia* (probably *C. phobifera*). Adult male flies gather at species-specific aggregation areas (e.g. hilltops that may be associated with man-made structures such as fire observation towers). Mating occurs with passing females, that are viviparous. White-tailed deer recognize the flies as irritants and display a range of specific avoidance behaviours. Female flies are attracted to increased concentrations of CO_2 and they lay larvae in the nasal cavity of the deer. First-stage instars are mainly found around the ethmoid bones, while second- and third-stage instars are found exclusively in the retropharyngeal area, which enlarges to form a pouch. Levels of infection per deer of 1–55 larvae, with an infection rate of 62%, have been recorded. Few clinical signs are associated with infection and infestation is not thought to have an effect at the population level. Occasional deaths associated with larval penetration of the cranial cavity have been reported, as well as neurological signs associated with aberrant migration to the auditory regions. The significance of deer avoidance behaviour as a stressor is not known. As infections are isolated to the head, cephenymiasis has no effect on the meat quality of hunter killed deer.

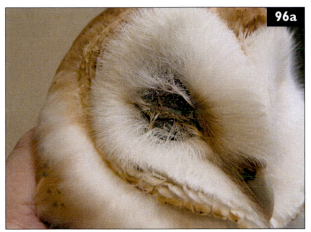

96 A barn owl is presented weak and thin and with extensive bruising around its right eye (96a).
i. What is the likely cause?
ii. What treatment should be given?

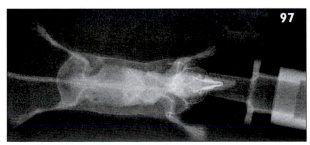

97 i. Identify the patient pictured in this ventrodorsal survey radiograph (97).
ii. What abnormalities do you see, and how might they have occured?
iii. Why is this presentation more common in birds?
iv. What treatment is indicated?

96 i. This is typical of a tick reaction to the bird tick *Ixodes frontalis*. There is intensive localized swelling around the head, with subcutaneous haemorrhage and tissue necrosis. The exact nature of the reaction is not known. Studies have not identified an infectious cause. Ticks attaching on the bird's body rather than the head rarely cause a reaction. Similarly, not all ticks stimulate a response (**96b** shows a tick on a common buzzard without reaction). It is possible that this is a toxin-related response or even a host–parasite incompatibility or anaphylactic response.

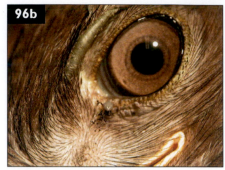

96b

ii. The bird will die without intervention. It should be given supportive care with fluid therapy (both systemic and oral) along with systemic antibiosis (e.g. amoxicillin or oxytetracycline). Corticosteroids (e.g. short-acting preparations of dexamethasone) are indicated, although these should be given with great care as they may themselves cause problems in birds. The prognosis is good provided therapy is given early and the bird is supported through treatment.

97 i. A shrew.

ii. The most obvious abnormality is a generalized subcutaneous emphysema. The skin is distended away from the body wall and there is a defect of the rib cage evident on the left thorax.

iii. Such injuries are most commonly produced following a cat attack, where the chest wall has been penetrated and air is able to leak from the lungs into the overlying tissues. Emphysema is more commonly seen in birds that have been caught by cats. The avian air sac system is extensive and particularly vulnerable to trauma. Both blunt trauma and penetrating injuries can cause air to leak from the air sacs into the subcutaneous tissues.

iv. Aggressive antibiotic cover is indicated where wounds are present, or indeed where the patient has been caught by a cat and no detectable wounds found. The inoculation of bacteria into a small mammal or bird following a cat bite or scratch will frequently lead to septicaemia and death. Broad-spectrum antibiotic cover is indicated as a mixed aerobic/anaerobic population has been recovered from the majority of cat bite wounds. A combination of clavulanate–amoxicillin and a fluoroquinolone is favoured, as fluoroquinolones on their own provide inadequate protection against anaerobic organisms and incomplete protection against *Streptococcus* spp.

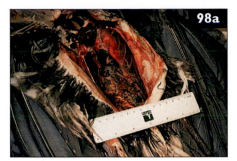

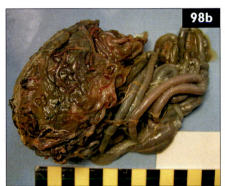

98 You are presented with a juvenile great blue heron that was found entangled in fishing line near the edge of a pond. You remove the line and the bird appears to be uninjured as a result. The bird is thin and has pale oral mucosae, but is otherwise bright and alert. The bird dies unexpectedly only a few hours later, so you conduct a post-mortem examination (98a–c).

i. What are the characteristic gross lesions that can be seen in 98a and 98b?
ii. What is the life cycle of the nematodes shown in 98c?
iii. Can these parasites be removed from a live bird?

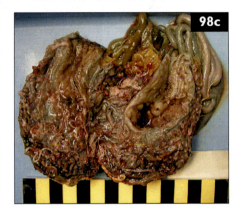

99 This deer (99) was diagnosed with chronic wasting disease (CWD) after being shot in southern Wisconsin, USA.
i. How is a diagnosis of CWD reached?
ii. What species are affected?
iii. Describe the clinical course of this disease.

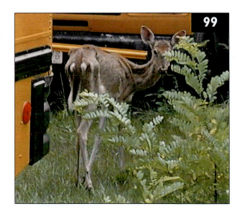

98 i. Parasitic tracts caused by the migration of the nematode *Eustrongyloides ignotus*.

ii. The larvae of *E. ignotus* are carried by fish ingested by herons. As the larvae develop into adult worms, they embed in the wall of the proventriculus and eventually migrate through the stomach wall into the coelomic cavity, causing a fibrinous reaction and coelomitis, as well as anaemia, emaciation and dehydration. The combination of the worms in the abdomen and the fibrinous reaction result in a 'ropey' feeling on palpation. The adults lay eggs within the migration tracts, which are carried back to the gastrointestinal (GI) lumen and expelled in the faeces, enter the water and are ingested by fish.

iii. If the worms have not caused too much damage, the bird can be treated systemically with ivermectin and long-term supportive care. If the damage is extensive, the GI tract will become non-functional and the bird will eventually die from direct damage to the GI tract or from secondary emaciation and anaemia.

99 i. Location should always be considered when assessing wildlife disease and CWD has been present in southern Wisconsin since late 2001. Diagnosis is by screening of retropharyngeal lymph nodes with an ELISA test and then confirmation of infection by immunohistochemical staining of the obex and the retropharyngeal lymph nodes for accumulation of CWD-associated prion protein.

ii. Wild and captive white-tailed and mule deer, rocky mountain elk, moose.

iii. In captive animals, subtle behavioural changes can precede more overt clinical signs. In wild animals, early signs may be difficult to recognize, but they may lead to an increased susceptibility to trauma, predation and hunting or exacerbate the effects of harsh winter environmental conditions. The clinical course in some deer has been characterized by acute death, with no noted clinical signs for over a year. The minimum incubation period in wild deer is thought to be 1.5 years. In the terminal stages, animals become emaciated (**99**), display abnormal behaviour, lose bodily functions and die. Signs in captive deer include excessive salivation, loss of appetite, progressive weight loss, hyperexcitability, tremors, excessive thirst and urination, listlessness, teeth grinding, holding the head in a lowered position and drooping ears. There are no distinctive gross pathological changes associated with CWD; however, aspiration pneumonia has been noted in some affected animals, presumably due to dysphagia and swallowing difficulties.

100 A young rabbit is found dead near a warren by a gamekeeper. It is in poor physical condition and on post-mortem examination you observe that there are several whitish, tortuous tracts beneath the liver capsule (**100a**). The gamekeeper has noticed similar lesions previously in cases he has examined and suspects tuberculosis.

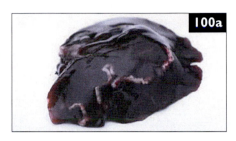

i. What would be your provisional diagnosis?
ii. What diseases would you include in your differential diagnosis?
iii. What tests would you carry out to establish a diagnosis?

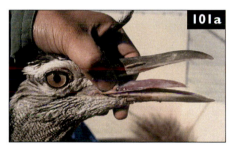

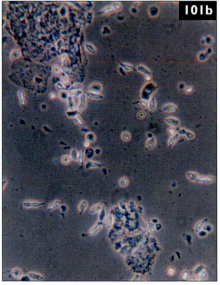

101 A male kori bustard from a flock that ranged freely in a large park was submitted for examination after it had been noted to be salivating excessively and inappetent. Physical examination findings included caseous lesions in the oropharynx, emission of foul odour from the mouth, emaciation, oral discharges and inflammation of the tongue (**101a**). A wet normal saline swab was examined directly using phase-contrast microscopy (400× magnification) (**101b**).

i. What is the diagnosis, and what are the differential diagnoses for oral lesions in birds?
ii. What is the route of infection?
iii. How would you treat this individual and prevent this disease causing problems in the flock?
iv. Why is this condition seasonal in some environments?

100 i. Hepatic coccidiosis caused by *Eimeria stiedae*.

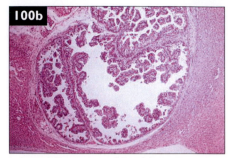

ii. The gross lesions may be confused with those of pseudotuberculosis caused by *Yersinia pseudotuberculosis* and of fascioliasis due to *Fasciola hepatica*. However, in yersiniosis the lesions are usually discrete caseous foci and in fascioliasis there is more severe and extensive fibrosis of the bile ducts. Neither condition is as common as hepatic coccidiosis in wild rabbits. Farmers, gamekeepers and hunters sometimes submit cases for laboratory examination believing the lesions are those of bovine tuberculosis.

iii. As a rapid test, place a bile sample on a glass slide and examine using a compound microscope. In most cases this will show large numbers of oocysts. Histopathological examination of liver will reveal remarkable hyperplasia of bile ducts, with the formation of large cystic spaces and massive numbers of coccidia developing in the epithelium (**100b**).

101 i. The saline swab reveals multiple flagellated protozoal organisms (*Trichomonas gallinae*) consistent with a diagnosis of trichomonosis. Differential diagnoses include diphtheritic pox, candidiasis, bacterial stomatitis and hypo-vitaminosis A.

ii. Transmission is by ingestion of contaminated food and water. Most species of pigeons are infected with *T. gallinae* and this bustard probably developed trichomonosis following indirect contact with food or water contaminated by infected birds.

iii. Bustards presented with early clinical signs respond well to metronidazole (50 mg/kg p/o q24h for 5–7 days). Cases with advanced lesions may need to be hospitalized. At-risk birds in 'closed' aviaries can be given preventive medication every 3–6 months. Birds in 'open' aviaries, where wild birds have access, should be given preventive medication every other month, alternating between dimetridazole and ronidazole. Dimetridazole has also been added to bustard pellets at a dose rate of 180 ppm as part of a preventive medicine programme.

iv. In the Middle East, a seasonal distribution of cases is observed. The highest prevalence is seen in the cooler months, while fewer cases occur during the hot summer months when the ambient temperature reaches its peak. This is because *Trichomonas* organisms are killed instantly on drying.

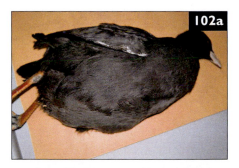

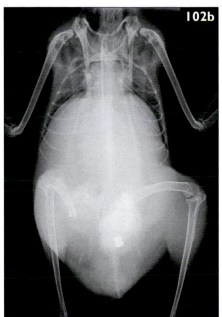

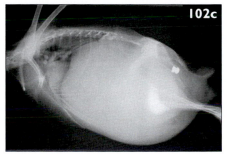

102 A coot was found by a member of the public and brought to a wildlife veterinary clinic. On clinical examination the bird was severely dyspnoeic and there was coelomic distension (102a).
i. What are the differential diagnoses in this case?
ii. Radiographs (ventrodorsal and lateral whole body views) were taken (102b, c). What do these show?
iii. What other tests would you perform as part of an initial diagnostic workup?
iv. What is the prognosis in this case?

103 You are presented with an orphaned but otherwise healthy badger cub of a few days old. What are the major considerations in the rearing and release of this animal?

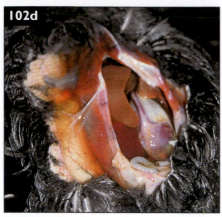

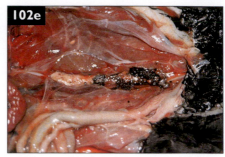

102 i. Egg binding peritonitis, organomegaly (hepatomegaly, renal enlargement, splenomegaly, etc), neoplasia, abscess, ascites, coelomitis.

ii. A metallic foreign body consistent with an air gun pellet is lodged within the caudal coelomic cavity. There is a general loss of coelomic visceral detail as well as a femoral fracture.

iii. Full blood count and serum biochemistry.

iv. Poor. The bird was euthanased and post-mortem examination revealed ascites (102d). The air gun pellet had tracked through the coelomic cavity, involving the left ovary and kidney (102e) and causing a severe coelomitis resulting from secondary bacterial infection from contaminants drawn in with the pellet.

103 Badger cubs require specialized facilities for successful rearing and release Warmth should be provided via an incubator or alternative heat source. Canine milk substitutes may be used, fed at rates and volumes similar to those used in puppies. Badger cubs do not naturally wean until they are 8–10 weeks old, so reasonably large cubs coming into captivity may still require bottle feeding. From eight weeks old, weaning foods such as breakfast cereals, scrambled eggs and minced meats can be introduced. Badger cubs require perineal stimulation to pass urine and faeces, usually after feeding. Badgers are social animals and orphaned cubs should be mixed with others of a similar age as soon as possible. Cubs reared as individuals have a tendency to develop abnormal behaviours and are not good candidates for release. As badgers are territorial, cubs cannot be released back into the area where they were found and must instead be released as new social groups in relatively badger-free areas with the landowner's full consent. Short-term artificial setts are constructed for this purpose. Cubs are released at 6–8 months old in groups consisting of more females than males and including at least two male animals.

104 What are the potential methods of euthanasia in stranded cetaceans?

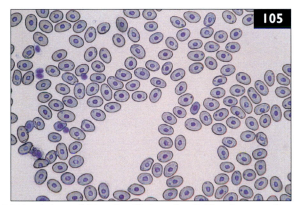

105 Around 95% of the red blood cells in a fresh blood smear from a green turtle contained these basophilic cytoplasmic inclusions (**105**).
i. What are these inclusions?
ii. Is this a normal finding?

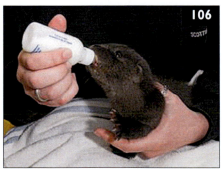

106 **i.** What is this species (**106**)?
ii. At what age can this orphaned, hand-reared animal be released into the wild?

104 Drug-induced euthanasia is the method of choice. Euthanasia using an intracardiac injection of pentobarbitone in a neonatal pilot whale is shown (104). Intravenous administration of pentobarbitone (60–200 mg/kg) is most frequently carried out using the central tail vessels in smaller species. Prior administration of a sedative (e.g. a benzodiazepine or alpha-2 agonist) is advisable. If intravenous administration proves difficult, pentobarbitone can be given via the intraperitoneal or intracardiac routes, using appropriate length needles.

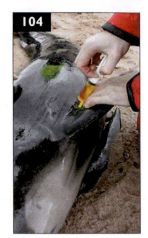

Etorphine hydrochloride (Large Animal Immobilon®) has also been used for cetacean euthanasia. Advantages include intramuscular administration and the relatively low volumes required (0.5 ml/1.5 metres in dolphins and porpoises and 4.0 ml/1.5 metres in whales). The major disadvantage is the serious risk to the operator and public safety. It is important to ensure appropriate disposal of the body to reduce risks to wildlife, domestic animals and the public.

If drugs are unavailable, stranded cetaceans up to 4 m in length can be shot, either through the blowhole at a 45° angle ventrocaudally to an imaginary line running through the pectoral fins, or via a shot aimed slightly up from just above the centre of the ear–eye line.

105 i. Cytoplasmic inclusion bodies.
ii. Although commonly confused with haemoparasites, cytoplasmic inclusion bodies in the red blood cells of green turtles are normal. They are also seen in other species of chelonia, such as the loggerhead sea turtle and the desert tortoise. They are degenerating organelles, appearing on electron microscopy as electron dense structures without any internal structure.

106 i. A Eurasian otter.
ii. Orphaned otter cubs that are hand reared should not be released until they are at least 12 months old. Wild otter cubs stay with and are dependent on their mother for a minimum of 12 months. During this time she shows them how to hunt, where the best feeding areas are and gets them fit enough to survive on their own. An otter cub reared in captivity must not be released if it is tame; it will not be able to fend for itself and will look for handouts from people. The best way to rear an otter cub is to have a 'hands off' approach and rear it with another otter of a similar age.

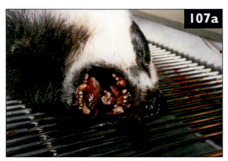
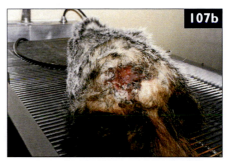

107 A local resident finds a badger hiding in the back of his garage. He is alerted to its presence by the attempts of his two dogs to attack it. He sees fresh blood on its nose and suspects that it might have involved in a road traffic accident (RTA) and then taken refuge. He is also concerned that his dogs have wounded the badger. There is no known badger sett in the vicinity. A local animal rescue group captures the animal and brings it in for examination. It is bright and aggressive and requires sedation for examination (107a, b).
i. What can you see, and what can you deduce about this badger?
ii. What advice can you give the local rescue group about the possibility of rehabilitation and release for this badger?
iii. What other factors would you take into consideration?

108 A mature female impala that had given birth the previous day was found with an everted swollen mass hanging through the vulval lips (108).
i. What is the diagnosis?
ii. What are the possible causes of this condition?
iii. What would be the treatment of choice if the organ was not necrotic?
iv. What are the potential complications associated with this condition and its treatment?
v. How would you treat this individual?

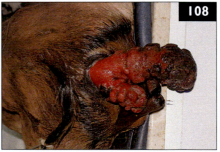

107 i. There appears to be some dried blood around the rhinarium, which may be consistent with a RTA, but the main observation is that there is marked attrition of the teeth, with severely worn or broken canines. The wound on the rump is of some long standing and is not due to an attack by dogs. This is a typical wound resulting from territorial fighting in badgers.

ii. This badger is almost certainly old and has been rejected from its sett. This will be the major reason it is hiding in human habitation. If rehabilitation and release is attempted, it is most likely that this badger will be attacked and driven out again, resulting in further injury and suffering. Therefore, the correct decision is euthanasia.

iii. Badgers are extremely territorial and should only be released back into the immediate area they came from. In some regions there is a high prevalence of tuberculosis in badgers and also a link between tuberculosis in badgers and cattle. Therefore, badgers should not be translocated without careful health screening and a thorough risk assessment. Tuberculosis is a zoonosis.

108 i. Post-parturient uterine prolapse. The exposed tissues are severely swollen and necrotic and in the early stages of putrification.

ii. The causes of this condition in wildlife are poorly documented. It is more prevalent in animals with a history of malnutrition and chronic disease.

iii. The uterus should be supported in an elevated position and kept clean. Calcium borogluconate should be administered and, if the animal is not anaesthetized, caudal epidural analgesia should be induced to eliminate straining. The exposed tissue should be cleaned, inspected for trauma (and for the presence of a distended bladder) and replaced according to techniques described for cattle. After reduction, oxytocin should be given. Vulval sutures may be required for 2–3 days to prevent recurrence.

iv. Haemorrhage, metritis, toxaemia, septicaemia, paresis, uterine rupture with bladder or intestinal eventration.

v. Amputation of the everted uterus. The procedure is performed under anaesthesia and comprises the application of an encircling ligature immediately behind the region of the cervix and subsequent excision of the prolapsed uterus about 8 cm posterior to the ligature. Amputation can be carried out with a scalpel blade or using cautery. Once the organ has been removed, the vagina and stump are replaced through the vulval lips into the pelvic canal. The prognosis is grave, since the risk of complications is high.

109 A common buzzard is admitted after being found on a road verge unable to fly and trailing one wing. Clinical examination reveals an emaciated juvenile with an open fracture of the right humerus. The wound appears to be fresh, with a sharp fragment of bone protruding through the skin. No other clinical abnormalities can be detected.

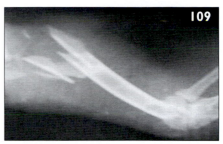

Palpation and radiography reveal a comminuted fracture with multiple fragments in the mid-third of the humerus (**109**). What is the prognosis, and what would you judge to be the best course of action?

110 A freshly dead, adult female wild hare was found at an equestrian property in February. It weighed 2.8 kg, was very lean and a post-mortem examination showed absence of internal body fat. The teeth and alimentary tract appeared normal and there was 65 g of food in the stomach. The spleen, adrenals and kidneys were all swollen. There was no pregnancy in the uterus, but the distal half of the left uterine horn was notably swollen. An adhesion extended from the left ovary to the site on the left uterine horn where the swelling started. The swollen horn (only) contained a mass of inspissated pus from which a profuse growth of *Staphylococcus aureus* was isolated (**110**). What are the two most likely contributions to the hare's chronic weight loss and eventual death?

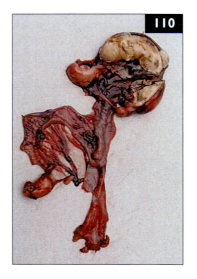

111 What factors affect the post-release survival rates of oiled birds?

109 Repair of a fractured avian humerus, especially to preserve accurately the anatomy and full function of the wing, is extremely difficult. This is due to the sigmoid shape of the humerus. Because the humerus is pneumatized, it possesses a thin cortex that easily shatters, forming sharp shards that frequently lacerate soft tissue structures and penetrate the skin, resulting in an open and potentially infected fracture site. For a rehabilitated avian casualty to survive in the wild it must have a near perfect ability to fly. The chance of success in this case is highly unlikely. Euthanasia would be the most humane course of action with, whenever possible, a full explanation of the rationale behind this decision being given to the finder of the casualty.

This is a frequent scenario. In their first year, juvenile buzzards may have difficulty finding food, lose body condition, become weak and, being carrion feeders, are attracted to road kills and hence fall victim to road traffic accidents. Such casualties, although directly associated with human activity, might well reflect the inability of the individual to survive in the wild and so, in reality, be a casualty of natural selection.

110 (1) Well established uterine sepsis, possibly the result of uterine trauma in the last pregnancy. The adhesion around the injured site may have prevented adequate drainage of infected material away from the distal half of the horn. (2) Secondary amyloidosis of spleen, adrenal and kidney, as in this case. The liver is also a site that often shows amyloid deposition.

Amyloidosis is a common observation in wild hares that have a chronically infected site. Even without treatment, if the site is small and the infection not life threatening, the hare survives the infection, but death results from the effects of secondary amyloidosis and not from the primary infection.

111 Survival rates vary depending on many different factors. These include the species of bird affected, the oil type spilt, weather conditions on release, facilities available for rehabilitation and length of time in captivity. Survival to release can be as high as 60%; however, post-release survival rates in auks are reportedly low. Other bird species, such as mute swans and jackass penguins, have higher post-release survival rates. The reason for this is unknown. It may be that inadequate food sources and immunosuppression are factors involved in lower post-release survival rates.

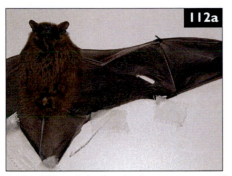
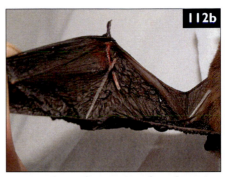

112 Wing injuries in bats are usually traumatic and may involve the wing membrane, the skeleton, or both of these structures. A small membrane tear as a result of a fishing hook injury, which did not impair the animal's flight, and a compound metacarpal fracture are shown (**112a, b**). What should be considered when assessing such injuries?

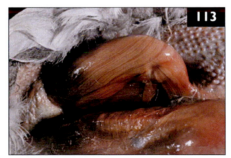

113 i. Which of the following are risk factors for the development of capture myopathy: prolonged chasing; struggling during restraint; capture in high or very low ambient temperatures; noisy surroundings during capture and handling; high humidity; pre-existing vitamin E deficiency; all of the above.
ii. Which of the following animals are considered to be at particularly high risk of development of capture myopathy: ungulates; primates; elephants; long-legged birds; big cats; birds of prey.
iii. When do signs of capture myopathy (affected muscle at post-mortem examination is shown; **113**) develop?
iv. What treatment should be given, and is it effective?
v. How can capture myopathy be prevented?

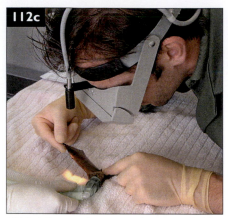

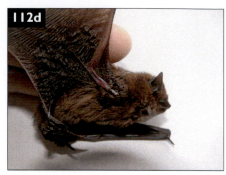

112 A thorough assessment of the full extent of any injury should be made. Use of magnifying lenses and good lighting (**112c**) is mandatory and many of these patients will benefit from a radiographic evaluation.

More extensive damage to wing membranes may significantly impair a bat's flying ability and this should be carefully evaluated prior to release. The majority of fractures of the wing are compound (humerus, **112d**) and these bats should be euthanased in view of the poor prognosis for such patients.

113 i. All of the above.
ii. Ungulates, long-legged birds.
iii. At any time from minutes after capture to days or weeks after the event.
iv. Fluid therapy with balanced electrolyte solution to counteract dehydration, hyperkalaemia, metabolic acidosis and myoglobinuria; sodium bicarbonate to resolve metabolic acidosis and to increase urinary pH; hyperbaric oxygen, if available (as used in human medicine); multivitamins (effectiveness unclear); benzo-diazepines to relax muscles and reduce stress; analgesia. Treatment is often ineffective, particularly in individuals with severe clinical signs.
v. Avoid catching in very high or low ambient temperatures or in high humidity. Minimize chasing. Ensure effective restraint by experienced personnel and minimize restraint times. Avoid prolonged restraint in unnatural positions (do not keep long-legged birds with their legs folded up). Minimize external stressor stimuli such as noise and sight of humans (use blindfolds); use capture drugs, which minimize induction and recovery times and promote physiological stability. Consider giving vitamin E supplementation in the period prior to capture and transport of known susceptible species.

114 Wildlife casualties are often found by members of the general public, who subsequently seek telephone advice from local veterinary practices regarding appropriate capture and handling of these animals. What specific advice on handling would you give to someone finding: (**1**) a raptor; (**2**) a hedgehog; (**3**) a fox?

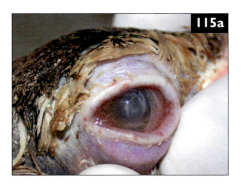

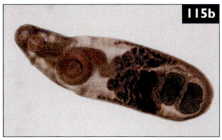

115 A free-ranging white-bellied bustard from a multispecies wildlife park in Dubai was caught up for examination after the keepers observed an ocular discharge (**115a**). Clinical examination revealed a severely inflamed conjunctiva with a villiform-like appearance of the surface of the conjunctival sac. A microscopic view of one of many parasites found on examination of a swab taken from the conjunctival sac is shown (**115b**).
i. Identify this parasite.
ii. What is the recommended treatment for this condition?
iii. What is the life cycle of this parasite?
iv. How do birds become infected with this parasite?

114 (1) Danger to handlers is possible from talons and beak. The handler should wear stout leather gloves. The whole bird should be covered with a thick blanket, cloth or coat, allowing the talons to grip the material and restrain the legs. Once captured, the bird should be picked up so the wings cannot be forced open. The bird may be carried this way for a short journey or placed in a darkened secure box with ventilation holes.

(2) Danger to handlers arises from scratches from the quills. This includes the possibility of ringworm infection. Hedgehogs should be picked up wearing thick gloves, a thick blanket or a coat through which quills cannot penetrate. A small, darkened, secure box with ventilation holes and bedding should be used for transportation.

(3) Foxes are dangerous animals and can cause severe bite injuries to handlers, so the general advice would be not to attempt handling. They should be handled only by experienced staff with appropriate equipment. Restraint of the head with a cat catcher or careful manual restraint of the scruff will allow transfer into a secure container (e.g. a wire crush cage darkened by covering with a blanket). In an emergency, a stout dustbin with a secure lid may be an alternative for transportation.

115 i. The eye fluke *Philophthalmus distomatosa*.

ii. Little has been published on the treatment of this condition. *P. gralli* have been physically removed from anaesthetized ostriches, with concurrent topical application of carbamate. Creoline has been used, applied directly into the eye of infested chicks following prior application of topical anaesthesia. Repeated doses of parenteral and topical doramectin and praziquantel have been attempted in bustards, but appear ineffective. The parasites can be removed manually under general anaesthesia using microforceps. Topical antibiotic eye drops should be administered because secondary bacterial infections are common.

iii. The life cycle of *Philophthalmus* spp. consists of birds as the final host and water snails as intermediate hosts. Larval stages have been found in the viviparous aquatic snail, *Melanoides tuberculata*, in the Middle East. Infected snails produce cercariae that form floating metacercarial cysts at the water surface.

iv. Following ingestion of metacercarial cysts when drinking.

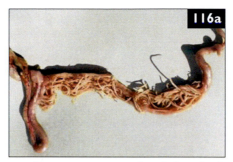

116 In early winter, an immature sparrowhawk is submitted for post-mortem examination. The muscular condition is very poor and the blood appears anaemic. The liver is shrunken and the gall bladder is distended with bile. The proventriculus is empty and there is only blackish mucoid material in the gizzard. The intestines are full of large nematodes (**116a**).
i. What is the likely primary problem?
ii. What lesions may have been missed on examination?
iii. What is the identity and significance of the nematodes?

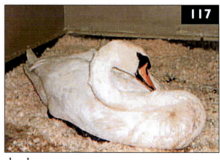

117 An adult mute swan is admitted to the practice in dry weather during the summer with profound weakness and unable to stand without support or fly (**117**). It is in reasonable body condition, has dirty ventral plumage and is attempting to 'walk' using its wings by flapping them into the ground, to the extent that it has superficially traumatized both carpi. At rest it is positioned with its head and neck laying on its body.
i. What are the most likely differential diagnoses for this case?
ii. What history taking, clinical examination and diagnostic procedures would you carry out?
iii. What action might it be useful to carry out in the environment from which the bird came?

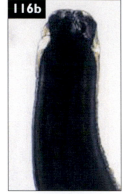
116b

116 i. Starvation. Sparrowhawks are predators of birds and do not feed on carrion, invertebrates or small mammals. Inexperienced sparrowhawks often find it difficult to kill sufficient prey.

ii. It is not uncommon in these cases to find that a wing joint, particularly a carpus, has been damaged and is swollen and/or inflamed. This is probably caused by a collision and although it may not be obvious on post-mortem examination, it is likely to have impaired the bird's hunting ability.

iii. *Porrocaecum depressum*, an ascarid-type worm commonly seen in the intestine of debilitated sparrowhawks. The head of a worm, with ascarid-type mouth parts, is shown (**116b**). Although they almost certainly develop as a consequence of malnutrition, heavy infections can occlude the gut and are therefore significant.

117 i. Botulism (*Clostridium botulinum* type C toxicity), lead poisoning or (less likely) any generalized systemic illness or trauma to the spine, pelvis or hindlimbs. Botulism is most likely, as this has a relatively rapid onset, although recent ingestion of a large amount of particulate lead is possible.

ii. It is important to know the site where the swan was found, what it was doing when found, how long it was there, and whether its condition has deteriorated since then. A full clinical and neurological examination should be carried out. Both lead poisoning and botulism produce generalized weakness and incoordination and 'limber neck', where the head and neck lie back across the body. Both conditions can occur at the same time of year, as lowered water levels expose lead and anaerobic silt. Botulism is often associated with diarrhoea, and lead poisoning with bright green faeces. Radiographic examination of the spine, pelvis, hindlimbs and ventriculus and blood lead analysis should be performed.

iii. Animals dying from botulism constitute a source of ingested toxin for other birds, particularly scavenging species such as gulls. Carcases should be removed, birds deterred from feeding from the area and, if possible, water flow and depth increased to remove and reduce access to the toxin.

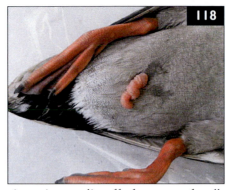

118 You are called to investigate a die-off of a group of mallards. You arrive at the wetland area and notice that several carcases have the clinical sign shown (118). In addition, several carcases have bloody fluid draining from the nares.
i. What is the most likely diagnosis?
ii. What gross pathological signs would you expect to see, and how would you confirm your diagnosis?
iii. What is the significance of this disease to free-ranging waterfowl populations?

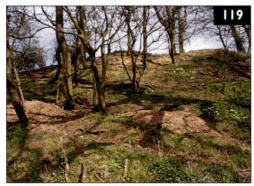

119 Active holes at a badger sett are shown (119). Badgers are social mammals and in the UK usually live in groups of 3–10 individuals, often occupying a well-defined territory. Badgers are implicated in the transmission of bovine tuberculosis to cattle. How might the social behaviour of badgers influence attempts to control the disease by means of vaccination or culling?

118 i. Duck viral enteritis (DVE) (also known as duck plague), which is caused by a herpesvirus. Clinical signs include loss of fear of humans, photophobia, reluctance to fly, convulsions and death. Birds may also have a blood-stained vent and a bloody discharge from the nares or mouth. Male birds will often have a prolapsed phallus (as illustrated).

ii. Petechial and ecchymotic haemorrhages on the heart, pinpoint necrotic foci in the liver, dark bands of haemorrhage and necrosis in the intestines of ducks (in geese these necrotic areas are circular), and necrotic plaques and pseudomembranes in the oesophagus. Confirmation is by isolation of the virus from sick or dead waterfowl. DVE infection may also be detected by PCR assay.

iii. There have been at least two extensive outbreaks of DVE in North America involving several thousands of birds. Wild waterfowl may or may not represent a significant natural reservoir for the virus. However, DVE has the potential to be detrimental to wild waterfowl populations and its periodic occurrence in captive or feral waterfowl should be contained or eliminated to avoid spillover into wild populations. Captive populations can be vaccinated against the virus. Minimizing other mechanisms by which DVE virus might be transferred into wild populations of waterfowl is also appropriate.

119 Some or all of the following important relationships should be considered. In much of the UK the organisation of badger populations into discrete social groups, occupying conspicuous setts, provides convenient units for targeting management efforts. Consequently, accurate information on the spatial distribution of badger setts is likely to be an important prerequisite for any such intervention. Vaccine delivery in the form of an oral bait would be facilitated by group aggregation, but deployment methods to ensure a sufficiently large proportion of the population took the bait would need to be developed. A further consideration would be frequency of bait deployment, which would partially depend on the rate of recruitment of susceptible animals to the population.

Intensive long-term studies suggest that a stable social structure may limit the spread of bovine tuberculosis in badger populations by reducing the extent of movement between social groups. This social stability, however, has been shown to break down in response to culling, resulting in increased levels of movement amongst badgers and potentially increasing the opportunities for contact with cattle. Culling may, therefore, may be associated with both positive and negative impacts on the incidence of tuberculosis in local cattle. It remains to be seen whether such effects are short lived or persistent.

120 A short-beaked echidna (**120**) has been hit by a car. The driver of the vehicle reported that the animal walked away from the incident apparently unharmed except for some bleeding from the head. The animal has since dug itself into the surface soil at the side of the road.

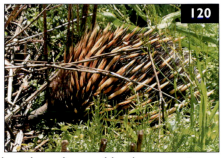

i. Describe how you would handle and restrain this animal to evaluate it further.

ii. Which bones, if any, are most likely to have been damaged by the trauma?

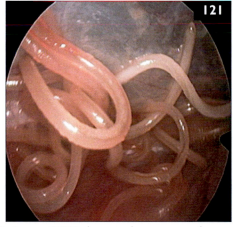

121 This endoscopic image (**121**) shows a large mass of roundworms in the lower respiratory tract of a wild saker falcon that had been confiscated from trappers and submitted for examination before release at a rehabilitation centre.

i. Identify the parasite.

ii. Is this infection significant in wild falcons, and should the bird be treated before release?

iii. If so, what is the treatment protocol?

iv. Are other birds at the rehabilitation centre at risk from infection? If so, how might the centre control this parasite?

120 i. It is virtually impossible to lift an echidna that has dug itself into the surface soil by sheer force. It is usually necessary to dig down beside the animal and push it up from below. Once freed from the soil, echidnas will roll themselves into a tight ball, but they can be handled with thick leather gloves. If the animal relaxes and a hindlimb is seen protruding, this limb can be grabbed and the animal held up in the air to permit at least a superficial examination of the body. To conduct a thorough examination, anaesthesia is usually necessary. The anaesthetic agent of choice is isoflurane. Induction in a chamber and maintenance via a mask is appropriate in most cases.
ii. The thick spines and significant subcutaneous fat layer of echidnas often protects the bulk of their body from trauma. However, the delicate maxilla and mandible within the beak are relatively unprotected and often damaged when these animals suffer vehicle-induced trauma. Fractures of these bones are often comminuted. The mouth and nasal cavity should, therefore, be carefully evaluated in any echidna trauma case.

121 i. *Serratospiculum* spp. Nine species are described in falcons. *S. seurati*, the most common species, is a large filarial worm found within the air sac membranes, visceral membranous serosa and connective tissue of the coelomic cavity of raptors.
ii. Field studies have shown that 10–15% of the wild saker falcon population in central Asia are infected with this parasite. It is also commonly found in wild peregrine and gyr falcons in central Asia and the former Soviet Union. Wild prairie falcons are commonly affected in the USA. Wild falcons are probably well adapted to this parasite, but opinions as to its pathogenicity in captive falcons vary. Some authors believe that *Serratospiculum* spp. infections can contribute to morbidity in wild-caught falcons that are used in falconry as part of stress-induced lower respiratory disease syndromes (e.g. aspergillosis or bacterial airsacculitis).
iii. Current treatment protocols include ivermectin or doramectin (0.2 mg/kg i/m weekly for 3 weeks). Many clinicians consider that heavy infestations of dead parasites should be removed endoscopically from the coelomic cavity.
iv. The life cycle of the parasite is indirect, with an arthropod as an intermediate host. Eradication of invertebrates (e.g. beetles) within the environment of raptor facilities is an important control measure.

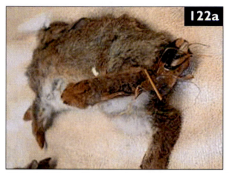 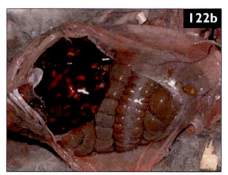

122 i. What disease should be suspected in wild weanling rabbits presenting with diarrhoea (**122a**) and hepatomegaly (**122b**)?
ii. What post-mortem findings and ancillary tests confirm this suspicion?
iii. What treatment options may be considered?

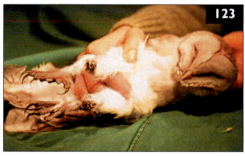

123 An adult male barn owl has been found in mid-summer caught in a 'pole' trap (a spring-trap placed on the top of an upright pole used illegally to control raptors). The bird is in good body condition and has fresh, open fractures to both tarsometatarsi (**123**). There appear to be no pedal reflexes.
i. What courses of action could be considered?
ii. The barn owl population in many places is in serious decline. This adult bird is likely to be feeding young. Does this affect any decisions?
iii. The use of such traps is illegal in some countries. What action should be taken in such circumstances?

122   i. Hepatic coccidiosis, caused by the rabbit-specific protozoan parasite *Eimeria stiedae*. Clinical symptoms may vary as a function of the severity of infection and the immune status of the individual. Signs include weight loss, ascites, jaundice, diarrhoea and hepatomegaly.

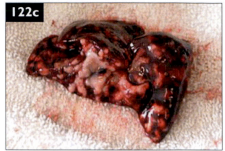

ii. Post-mortem signs reflect this parasite's predilection for the bile ducts. The gallbladder and bile ducts are likely to be thickened and distended (**122c**). The swollen gallbladder may be sampled and wet bile smears made to reveal large numbers of coccidial oocysts. Raised serum bilirubin levels in young rabbits are virtually pathognomic for hepatic coccidiosis. Elevated AST, ALKP, GGT and ALT readings may also be seen.

iii. A number of anticoccidial drugs, including sulphaquinoxaline, toltrazuril and robenidine, have been used to treat *E. stiedae*. Treatment failure is to be expected where oral medication is supplied to inappetent or anorectic rabbits. Such rabbits may be best euthanased. Response to treatment can be good when sulpha drugs are administered to rabbits that are active and eating well. Newly weaned animals that recover from hepatic coccidiosis possess lifelong immunity from the disease. Diclazuril (4 mg/kg single s/c injection) has been shown to be effective in controlling clinical coccidiosis in rabbits.

123 i. In the absence of complications (infection/soft tissue damage), such fractures respond well to immobilization using external fixation. However, this case appears to involve soft tissue damage and, as both legs are fractured, the bird would need support in the form of a sling, which might prove to be very stressful or, indeed, impracticable. Euthanasia would be the more humane approach.

ii. The welfare of the bird must be the first consideration. Although the male is the primary provider of food for the brood, the female is still likely to be capable of providing for some of the young, at least. If the nest site is known, then supplementary food can be given. Even if treatment was successful, the young would have fledged by the time the injured bird could be released and, depending on the local barn owl population, it is likely that another male would rapidly fill his place.

iii. Cases of illegal use of traps should be reported to the appropriate authorities.

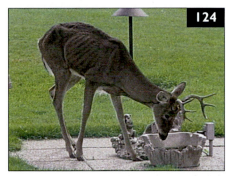

124 i. What abnormalities are present in this white-tailed deer (**124**).
ii. Provide a list of differential diagnoses.

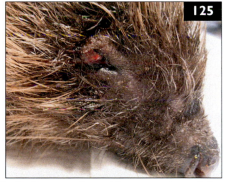

125 This European hedgehog was found by a member of the public out during the day time with extensive lesions (**125**).
i. Describe your approach to this patient.
ii. What is the prognosis in this case?

126 A long-term captive grey squirrel is presented with weight loss, polydipsia and lethargy. The squirrel is in good condition, weighs 750 g and is eating well. Urinalysis shows a high urine glucose concentration, ketonuria and a SG of 1.010.
i. What condition would you consider likely, and what may have predisposed the animal to this?
ii. How might this condition be treated?

124 i. The signs are not specific for any particular disease aetiology. This deer is emaciated as assessed by prominence of the ribs and pelvic bones. White-tailed deer are generally crepuscular/nocturnal, suggesting behavioural change, as does the close proximity to human structures.

ii. Trauma (animals survive with fractures that heal by secondary intention after encounters with hunters); chronic wasting disease; systemic spread of localized abscesses (gunshot, arrow or fight wounds; 'cranial abscess syndrome'); *Mycobacterium bovis* infection; rabies; *Mycobacterium paratuberculosis* subsp. *avium*; *Baylisascaris procyonis* infection; malnutrition (more likely to manifest under harsh winter conditions); chronic bronchopneumonia; dental disease; tooth wear in an aged animal; foreign body obstruction; severe endoparasitism.

125 i. As with all wildlife, an initial brief physical examination is performed to permit triage of the patient. In general, hedgehogs should not be active during the day and if the lesions observed have just occurred, it is likely disease other than the recent trauma is present. Once the extent of the pathology has been determined, the prognosis will be known and a decision can be made on whether to treat or euthanase the animal.

ii. Hedgehogs commonly survive quite severe infections, and limb fractures may be treated using fixation or amputation. Supportive care should be administered. This animal had extensive lesions, including avulsion of the right eye (likely due to head trauma), and it was unresponsive to stimuli. It was euthanased on welfare grounds without further investigation or treatment.

126 i. The urine test results are highly suggestive of diabetes mellitus. Despite the recent weight loss, this animal is overweight (normal average 500–600 g). Grey squirrels in captivity often gain weight through inappropriate feeding and sedentary life styles. In other mammalian species this is known to predispose to diabetes mellitus (in particular type II diabetes).

ii. Diabetes may be treated by administration of regular insulin injections and monitoring of blood glucose. This was considered both impractical and stressful in this case. An alternative treatment is diet modification and oral hypoglycaemic drugs (sulphonylurea drugs, alpha-glucosidase inhibitors or biguanides). This squirrel was treated with the sulphonylurea drug glipizide (0.5–1 mg/kg p/o q12h), together with a controlled low-sugar diet. Urine glucose and ketone levels were monitored on a weekly basis and doses of glipizide adjusted until the urine was free of ketones and glucose levels had reduced.

There are no known reports of diabetes in squirrels, but the author has successfully treated three captive squirrels in this way. The presence of concurrent endocrinopathies, such as hyperadrenocorticism or thyroid disorders, should also be considered.

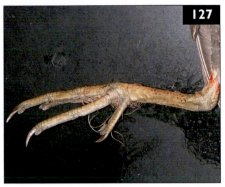

127 A moorhen is presented to your practice as shown (**127**).
i. What would your course of action be?
ii. What short-term environmental requirements would you have to provide for this animal?
iii. What wider action might you take after seeing this case?

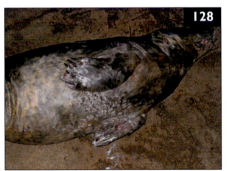

128 You are called to see a four-month-old grey seal at a newly set up marine wildlife rehabilitation facility (**128**). It has a number of inflamed lesions on the ventral thorax and abdomen, the palmar surfaces of the foreflippers and around the mouth. It is one of eight similarly aged grey seals at the facility, either in individual or shared cubicles. The plan is to transport them to a larger facility once they require greater pool space.
i. What is this condition, and why has it affected the seal in this manner?
ii. What is the prognosis for this animal?

127 i. After initial stabilizing treatment, the bird should be anaesthetized, all visible line removed and the bird examined for further line. Monofilament nylon can be drawn tightly around the extremities and cut into the skin without being immediately visible. Any circular wounds should be probed with a hypodermic needle or number 11 scalpel blade to locate and cut line in one place only, then the free ends grasped with fine forceps and unravelled. Fishing line may be associated with fishing hooks embedded in the skin or with line, hooks and weights in the gastrointestinal tract, although the latter is not common in this species. Survey radiography is recommended. It is advisable to monitor the animal for 48–72 hours following line removal to ensure vascular viability of the distal limb.

ii. Moorhens are easily stressed and should be kept out of sight and hearing of predatory species and humans. A quiet room, a partial cage covering and a 'hide' (e.g. cardboard box) are advised. Moorhens are predominantly piscivorous, but also eat snails, worms, seeds and berries. Finely chopped fish, worms, snails and insectivorous bird food may be provided, but they may not eat in captivity. Gavage with a diluted canine convalescent diet may be required, although this is stressful in itself.

iii. Encourage fishermen to retrieve fishing waste.

128 i. Seal pox, which predominantly affects grey seals rather than common or harbour seals, and mainly affects naïve juveniles. It is extremely infectious between seals and via fomites, mainly affecting the flippers, ventrum and mouth, all areas that come into contact with the floor and feeding utensils and are subject to small breaks in the skin. The widespread and moderately severe nature of the clinical appearance may be a result of immune suppression due to other diseases, malnutrition or secondary bacterial infection. The ventral thoracic spread is less typical and may, alternatively, reflect poor environmental hygiene.

ii. Good. Cases such as this may have some difficulty feeding due to the lesions around the mouth, and they may be in some discomfort due to the inflamed and ulcerating nature of the lesions. Uncomplicated cases with limited lesions, no secondary infection and minimal ulceration and bleeding hardly affect the animal and have an excellent prognosis. Very widespread lesions may reflect a poor underlying health status. Generally, affected individuals can be expected to improve over 4–8 weeks, with lesions healing and shrinking. Some lesions, especially on the lips and between the digits, may become infected with opportunistic environmental bacteria and generate a purulent discharge.

129 What would be your advice to the manager of the rehabilitation facility where the grey seal in **128** was kept?

130 An anaesthetized free-ranging mountain gorilla is shown (**130**). What is the most common reason for veterinary intervention in free-ranging mountain gorillas?

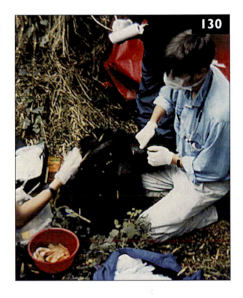

131 A dorsal view of the rump of an adult male badger, taken under general anaesthesia in January as part of a badger capture–mark–recapture study in the UK, is shown (**131**).
i. Describe the lesion seen.
ii. What is the likely aetiology?
iii. Discuss its behavioural and epidemiological significance.

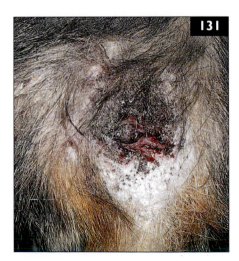

131

129 The seal should be treated with NSAIDs to reduce inflammation and discomfort and with long-acting broad-spectrum antibiotics (ideally in feed, but by parenteral injection if the animal is reluctant to eat). Cefovecin has been used in a small number of seals where antibiosis is essential, but repeated injection or oral medication has not been practical. The seal should be isolated and barrier nursed to avoid spread to other seals. It may be acceptable to allow other seals to be exposed to this infection at some stage, but not seals that are extremely young, systemically ill or debilitated, or otherwise immune suppressed. Environmental hygiene should be improved to avoid high environmental bacterial loads. A salt water environment may be beneficial in this respect. Infected lesions may be bathed in antiseptic solutions. Lesions that proliferate and bleed readily at the slightest trauma may benefit from surgical resection or cautery. Seal pox has very occasionally been reported to affect humans, so the use of latex gloves and meticulous hygiene is advised. Immunosuppressed humans and those with breaks in the skin on their hands and forearms should not handle affected animals.

130 Mountain gorillas will occasionally become ensnared in rope or wire snares that are set by poachers to capture forest ungulates. These snares will tighten around a wrist or ankle, act like a tourniquet and result in the loss of a hand or a foot, which could subsequently jeopardize the survival of this individual. Prompt removal of the snare is therefore essential to prevent the loss of an appendage. This particular gorilla was immobilized to remove a snare from the left wrist. She had already lost her left foot as a result of a previous snare injury.

131 i. There is an extensive area of hair loss over the rump, associated with a large purulent wound, matted with hair and tissue exudate.
ii. A bite wound from another badger.
iii. Bite wounds are not uncommon in badgers and tend to be more frequent and more severe in males than in females. Aggressive encounters between individuals may occur both within and between social groups, and in males they are probably associated with territorial disputes and reproductive competition. This study population is known to be infected with *Mycobacterium bovis*, the causal agent for bovine tuberculosis. Isolation of *M. bovis* bacilli from bite wounds is well documented, and has also been associated with rapid and progressive infection, leading to the hypothesis that bite wounds represent a potential route of disease transmission between badgers.

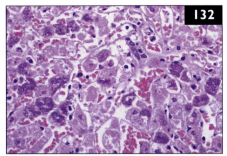

132 A large mature male hare (2.7 kg) was found dead. It had no signs of external trauma, discharges or diarrhoea and had no palpable abdominal impaction. At post-mortem examination there were plentiful internal fat deposits and 65 g of food in the stomach. The liver had a very prominent lobular pattern, the distended bladder contained dicoloured urine and the tracheal mucosa was intensely congested. Histological examination of the liver revealed a severe diffuse hepatopathy with necrosis of hepatocytes, some containing a basophilic stippling (**132**).

i. What is the diagnosis?
ii. Is this condition likely to affect rabbits?
iii. How frequently does it cause hare mortality?

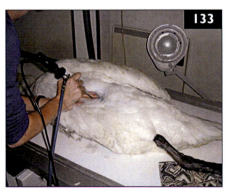

133 i. What are the three species of swan seen in the UK?
ii. Which species is a resident?
iii. What are common options for anaesthetic induction agents in large swans?
iv. What are the main indications for endoscopy (**133**) in swans?
v. What is the preferred site of entry for coelomic cavity examination?

132 i. European brown hare syndrome (EBHS), which is caused by a calicivirus. It was confirmed by electronmicroscopy in this case. The nature of the pathology and the fact that hares are usually in good bodily condition, but with a full stomach, when found dead, indicate that it is of sudden onset.
ii. EBHS does not cause disease in rabbits. (Rabbits can suffer from rabbit haemorrhagic disease, which is a lethal calicivirus infection.)
iii. In both hare and rabbit populations these caliciviruses can cause high mortality in a susceptible population. EBHS outbreaks have been reported every few years, but sometimes only a single case is found at a location.

133 i. Mute swan, Bewick's swan, Whooper swan.
ii. Mute swan.
iii. Mask induction is not generally practical in swans due to their size, so intravenous induction agents are generally used (e.g. 9 mg/kg ketamine plus 10 µg/kg medetomidine or 0.2 mg/kg xylazine i/v).
iv. Diagnostic laparoscopy and hook removal. Swans often show quite subtle signs of diseases such as aspergillosis. Overt respiratory signs are usually not evident. Endoscopy to visualize the air sacs and internal organs can be part of a general diagnostic workup for a bird that is not responsive to medical therapy. Some hooks in the oesophagus and proventriculus can be removed using a flexible endoscope with an instrument channel, avoiding the requirement for a proventriculotomy.
v. The swan is placed in right lateral recumbancy and the left leg pulled back to expose the caudal ribcage. The incision site is identified between the last two ribs, ventral to the spine and cranial to the femur. A small skin incision is made and the muscles between the ribs dissected bluntly using artery forceps. Entry into the air sacs is confirmed by an audible 'pop'. A rigid endoscope can then be placed into the coelomic cavity via this incision. There is no need to suture the wound postoperatively.

134 A black-headed gull is presented with a damaged wing. Examination reveals a bird in good body condition. Palpation and radiography indicate a closed fracture of the distal third of the radius (134a). No other obvious clinical abnormalities are found. What is the prognosis, and what would you judge to be the best course of action?

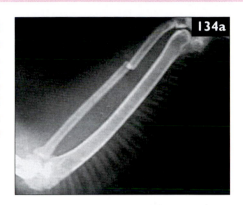

135 The Houbara bustard is listed in Appendix 1 of the Convention on International Trade in Endangered Species of Wild Fauna and Flora (CITES). These wild-caught birds are often smuggled from Pakistan into Middle Eastern countries, where they are used by falconers to train their falcons (135).

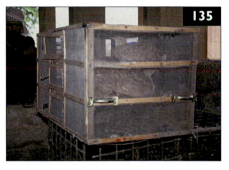

i. If these birds are discovered by customs officials at a port of entry, what is the appropriate action for the authorities to take?

ii. What disease considerations are there for birds that have been trafficked through markets, and why should falconers not consider these to be suitable birds to train their falcons?

iii. What problems should be considered if these birds are sent to a rehabilitation programme for release back into the wild or for incorporation into a captive breeding project?

iv. What issues might be of concern even if the birds are medically screened and determined to be healthy for potential release back into the wild?

134   Closed fractures of the ulna or radius usually have a good prognosis. The intact bone splints the fractured bone and, as long as the fragments are in at least partial apposition, stabilization of the fracture can occur within ten days and healing be complete within 3–4 weeks. Initially, the damaged wing will droop and, to prevent damage to the flight feathers, the wing can be supported with adhesive tape (ideally

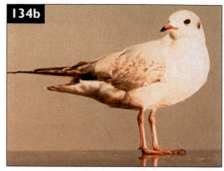

masking or autoclavable tape, as the adhesive used is unlikely to damage feathers, 134b). The tape is applied around the primaries and secondaries of the closed wing. Such support should not be left in place for periods of >5–7 days without being removed and the wing manipulated to prevent contraction of the tendons, which will lead to permanent restriction of joint mobility. Gulls with disabilities do not usually require special husbandry or feeding and they settle well in captivity. The disability is short term, requiring minimal interference. The casualty is quickly restored to normality and, where practicable, can be returned to the locality where it was found. In such a case there are few concerns regarding welfare.

135   i. If the country is a signatory to CITES, the government has to confiscate the birds.
ii. Smuggled birds have potentially been exposed to infectious agents, such as avian influenza, Newcastle disease and avian pox, during their shipment. There is a potential risk to falcons if trafficked birds are used as 'bagged' quarry to train them.
iii. These birds represent a potential disease risk to captive breeding programmes and free-living Houbara bustard populations if health monitoring and medical treatment are not instigated There is also a potential economic threat should these birds come into contact with local poultry flocks.
iv. There are IUCN Guidelines for the Placement of Confiscated Animals. Confiscated birds have often been moved a great distance from the site of capture; therefore, because the site of original capture of smuggled birds is unknown, it is difficult to establish an appropriate site for release that takes into account the biological and ecological needs of the individuals, the animal's genetic make-up and other aspects that are important to minimize risks (e.g. territorial competition) to free-living populations.

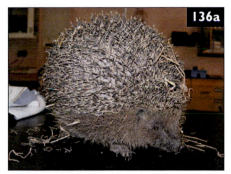

136 An adult male hedgehog, found by the side of a road, appears to be grossly inflated (**136a**). Although very large and round, it feels lighter than expected and the skin is spongy when pressed. It has some blood around the nose and one eye, and laboured breathing.

i. What is your diagnosis?

ii. How would you confirm the diagnosis?

iii. Why is this condition so dramatic in the hedgehog?

iv. What is the treatment and prognosis for such hedgehogs?

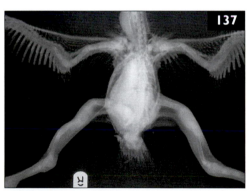

137 A juvenile Bonelli's eagle that had been removed from its nest in the wild and hand reared was presented for examination because it had drooping wings and was unable to stand. The bird was anaesthetized and radiographed (**137**).

i. What observations can you make from this radiograph?

ii. What is the condition affecting this bird?

iii. What are the causes of this condition?

iv. What free-living species has this condition been reported in?

136 i. Generalized subcutaneous emphysema ('balloon syndrome').

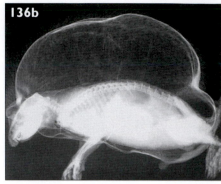

136b

ii. Needle aspiration will confirm the presence of air under the skin. Radiography can be used to support the diagnosis (**136b**).

iii. As a defence mechanism, hedgehogs have developed the ability to curl up tightly by contracting the strong purse string-like *orbicularis* muscle. In order to achieve curling, the dorsal skin is quite loose fitting, with a large potential subcutaneous space. Injury to the respiratory system can result in a large volume of air leaking under the skin and inflating the hedgehog. Such injuries are usually sustained in road traffic collisions and include rib fracture, airway penetration or tearing of the cranial mediastinum at the thoracic inlet. Rarely, the subcutaneous emphysema is caused by a gas-producing bacterial infection of a deep wound.

iv. Broad-spectrum antibacterial therapy and alleviation of the respiratory distress with oxygen therapy if required. Repeated deflation with stab incisions or needle aspiration may also be beneficial. The prognosis depends on the severity of the initial trauma and extent of other injuries (including pulmonary emphysema and haemorrhage). Many affected individuals do make a full recovery.

137 i. A generalized lack of density in the cortex of all the long bones. Folding fractures can be seen in the tibiotarsal, humerus, femur, radius and ulna bones.

ii. Severe metabolic bone disease.

iii. Metabolic bone disease encompasses a number of conditions that develop as a result of prolonged deficiencies of calcium or vitamin D_3 or of an improper dietary Ca:P ratio (normal ratio 1:1 to 2:1). Vitamin D deficiency can occur secondary to insufficient exposure to UVB light. Calcium deficiency leads to nutritional secondary hyperparathyroidism in raptor chicks. Adequate levels of both calcium and phosphorus are present in the natural diet of wild raptors because the bones and tissues of prey animals contain the correct Ca:P ratio. Metabolic bone disease occurs when birds are not offered a complete or balanced diet in captivity. This bird was being fed a meat-only diet.

iv. Wild collared doves, grey herons and young crows. In Africa, vulture chicks have been reported with metabolic bone disease, which has been attributed to a lack of calcium intake.

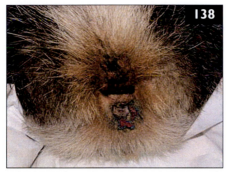

138 Injured European badgers found on the roadside may demonstrate blue-green colouration of their faeces (**138**). What should be suspected in such cases, and how can this be investigated further?

139 What documentation is available to guide those undertaking translocation of wildlife species?

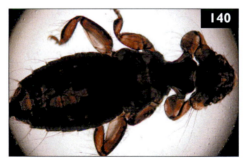

140 An invertebrate removed from the feather of a mute swan is shown (**140**).
i. What is this?
ii. What is its significance?

138 It must not be assumed that a badger found by the roadside has been hit by a car. Some may have been poisoned, have territorial fight wounds or be generally debilitated. Displaced individuals with territorial fight wounds are often hit by cars. There are a number of blue-coloured materials that badgers may ingest. Many products are coloured to aid identification (e.g. various food dyes are added to rodenticides and pesticides by manufacturers); however, there is no universal colouring code. Slug bait, containing methiocarb or metaldehyde, is also often coloured blue. Badgers are often subject to bait marking studies where coloured plastic can be mixed with peanuts and treacle. Badgers like peanuts and treacle and this combination appears to be commonly used as a vehicle for poisons for badgers. The presence of blue peanuts is therefore strongly suggestive of a deliberate attempt to poison.

History, clinical examination and other observations will help to ascertain a suspected diagnosis. Analysis of the bait is only likely to provide retrospective confirmation of the poison involved. In cases of suspected poisoning, stabilizing the patient and delivering symptomatic treatment is paramount. Further absorption of the toxicants must be prevented and efforts made to promote their speedy elimination.

139 Translocation planning is essentially an exercise in risk assessment. Three documents are available that guide those undertaking translocations:
- IUCN (1998) Guidelines for Re-Introductions. Prepared by the IUCN/SSC Re-Introduction Specialist Group, Gland, Switzerland and Cambridge, UK. 10 pp.
- IUCN Position Statement. Translocation of Living Organisms (1987).
- Woodford, MH (2000) (Ed) *Quarantine and Health Screening Protocols for Wildlife Prior to Translocation and Release into the Wild*. Published jointly by the IUCN Species Survival Commission's Veterinary Specialist Group, Gland, Switzerland, the Office International des Epizooties (OIE), Paris, France, Care for the Wild, UK, and the European Association of Zoo and Wildlife Veterinarians, Switzerland.

140 i. A feather louse, *Trinoton anserinum.*
ii. Small numbers are not usually associated with clinical signs, but large numbers of this biting louse may occur in debilitated swans that are not preening. In birds with a high burden, feather quality may be affected. This louse also serves as an intermediate host in the life cycle of the filarial heartworm (*Sarconema eurycerca*), causing disease in swans and geese.

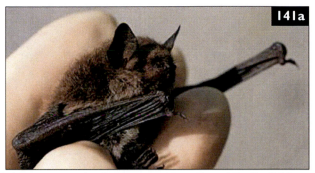

141 A UK fisherman caught this bat accidentally while fly fishing (**141a**). It bit him as he was unhooking it, but then died. There were no obvious external lesions and the bat was in good condition.
i. How should you proceed?
ii. Can you identify the species of bat, and what is the significance of this?

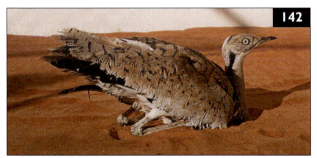

142 A wild adult male Houbara bustard was caught in a noose snare in order to fit satellite telemetry as part of a migration study for a conservation project. The bird was unable to stand or fly off when it was released and was retained in captivity for further veterinary investigation (**142**).
i. What condition is this wild bird suffering from based on the clinical signs observed and the history?
ii. What diagnostic samples might be useful to support the provisional diagnosis made?
iii. What are the differential diagnoses of this paresia in captive adult bustards?

141 i. The fisherman should be advised to seek medical attention immediately. If he has not already done so, the bite wound should be thoroughly washed with soap and water. In the UK, the relevant government agency should be advised of the incident and arrangements made to submit the bat for rabies testing.

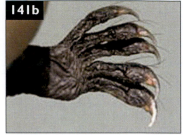

ii. The bat is a Daubenton's and all recorded cases of bat rabies (European bat lyssavirus) in the UK so far have been in this species. Daubenton's bats often feed by flying low over water and are occasionally caught by fly fishermen. They have unusually large feet with long hairy toes (**141b**), which are used to take food items from the surface of water.

142 i. Capture myopathy or capture paresis.

ii. In addition to haematology, heparinized blood samples should be collected for biochemical analysis. Diagnosis is based on consideration of the history, clinical signs and detection of elevated plasma levels of creatine kinase (CK), aspartate aminotransferase and lactate dehydrogenase. Elevation of serum CK concentration appears to be the most sensitive and specific index of muscle damage in both mammals and birds.

iii.

- Traumatic causes: vertebral fractures or luxations, multiple fractures, pelvic fractures, dislocations, sprains.
- Infectious causes: neuritis (peripheral nerve), encephalitis or encephalomyelitis, intervertebral abscess, septicaemia with spinal infection, nephritis, viral infections (PMV group, reovirus), bacterial infections (e.g. *Chlamydophila* spp., *Listeria* spp., *Yersinia* spp., *Salmonella* spp., *Streptococcus* spp.), fungal infections (aspergillosis involving the central nervous system).
- Metabolic/nutritional causes: vitamin E/selenium deficiency.
- Reproductive causes: obturator paralysis following difficult egg delivery, egg binding, broken leg from calcium deficiency, ectopic eggs.
- Neoplastic causes: renal adenocarcinoma, fibrosarcoma, other neoplasia or space-occupying lesion (e.g. haematoma).
- Poisons: botulism, lead toxicosis, ionophore toxicity.
- Miscellaneous causes: cloacal lithiasis.

143 List the post-release monitoring options for rehabilitated seal pups.

144 i. Describe the condition this adult male eastern bearded dragon is suffering from (**144**).
ii. What are the possible causes of this condition?
iii. How would you treat it?

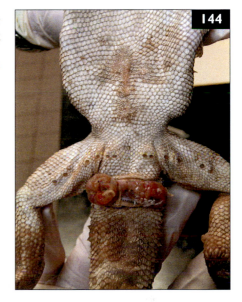

145 This swan was rescued from the wild by a member of the public and brought to the veterinary surgery for further assessment and treatment. On clinical examination you notice the lesions shown (**145**).
i. What species is this?
ii. What sex is this swan, and how can this be determined?
iii. What is this likely cause of the injuries seen, and what is the prognosis in this case?

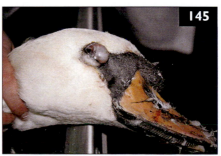

143 Hind flipper rototags (143), head tags and satellite relay data loggers.

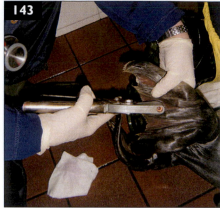

143

144 i. Bilateral hemipene prolapse.
ii. Blunt trauma to the lumbosacral region or trauma to the hemipene itself during mating can cause swelling and an inability to retract the organ/s into the associated pocket. The condition may also be seen secondary to infection of the reproductive structures or generalized weakness.
iii. The prolapsed tissue should be properly identified and tissue viability assessed prior to any attempt at repair. If viable, the exposed tissue can be soaked in hypertonic saline (to reduce oedema), then flushed with sterile saline, lubricated and gently replaced. Surgical débridement may be necessary if the tissue is damaged or necrotic. Holding sutures can be placed temporarily at the opening to the hemipene pocket to prevent immediate re-prolapse. The animal should be thoroughly evaluated for concurrent disease. Body and scale condition in this individual is suboptimal, suggesting that there may be other contributing health concerns.

145 i. A mute swan.
ii. A male (cob). Males are larger and weigh more on average than females (called pens). During the breeding season the fleshy area above the nares enlarges and becomes engorged in the male. This area is often termed 'the knob'. Outwith the breeding season it is more difficult to tell the sexes apart.
iii. Injuries to the head are often caused by territorial fighting between rival swans during the breeding season. Fierce territorial combats in which the dominant male uses his wings to beat against the opponent are common. This bird has severe ocular traumatic injuries involving both eyes and therefore its prognosis for return to the wild is poor. The loss of one eye may be well tolerated and is often seen in wild swans apparently coping well with this disability; however, complete loss of sight has an extremely poor prognosis.

146 A European badger has been brought to your veterinary practice suffering from injuries caused by a road traffic accident (RTA).
i. What are the potential zoonotic disease risks from this animal?
ii. What safety precautions should be taken to minimize risks to staff?
iii. Outline your approach to this case.

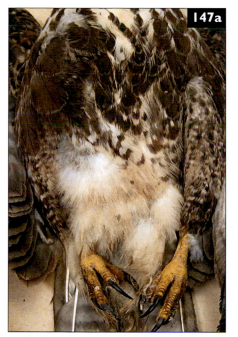

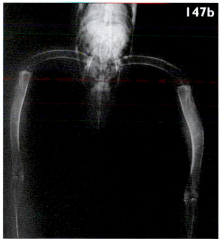

147 The legs of a sub-adult common buzzard that was hit by the author's car are shown (**147a**). It died almost immediately after. A ventrodorsal radiograph of the bird was taken (**147b**).
i. What do you notice about the legs?
ii. What does the radiograph demonstrate, and does it confirm your suspicions from examination of the bird?

146 i. If thoracic penetration has occurred, badgers with tuberculous pulmonic lesions are a significant source of infection for human carers. *Leptospira* spp. and *Salmonella* spp. have been isolated from badgers. Badgers are also susceptible to anthrax. Sarcoptic mange has been reported in Europe.

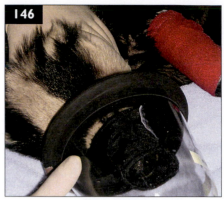

ii. Badgers are dangerous animals; care should be taken to avoid being bitten (e.g. use basket or nylon fabric muzzles designed for dogs). Gloves should be worn during examination of the animal, and hygiene measures undertaken. Facemasks are advisable, particularly if draining abscesses are present. Unless the animal is comatose, examination is usually performed under general anaesthesia (e.g. medetomidine 20 µg/kg with ketamine 4 mg/kg and butorphanol 0.4 mg/kg administered i/m). The muzzled badger shown (**146**) is receiving oxygen by inhalation mask.

iii. Animals that survive the initial trauma following a RTA will be suffering from shock. Initial first aid (e.g. subcutaneous fluids, analgesia) should be provided to stabilize the patient before sedation or anaesthesia. Common injuries include fractures, thoracic trauma and abdominal trauma. A thorough assessment includes a clinical examination and thoracic and abdominal radiographs. Further diagnostics (e.g. ultrasonography, haematology, biochemistry) may be appropriate. Badgers do not adapt well to hospitalization and this often limits feasible treatments. If severe injuries are detected or tuberculosis is suspected, the animal should be euthanased.

147 i. There is bowing, especially of the tibiotarsal bones.

ii. Lesions typical of osteodystrophy due to nutritional secondary hyperparathyroidism ('rickets'). This has almost certainly occurred secondary to the abundance of road kill carrion found along that road that year. This will result in overfeeding of the young by the parent birds and hence selective feeding of muscle rather than bone. While the bone changes were unlikely to have been responsible for the bird's behaviour in flying near the road, they would certainly have been factors that would have made this bird less likely to survive a harsh winter. This case illustrates the need to examine the whole bird and not just concentrate on acute injuries and their healing before making the decision to release a bird back to the wild.

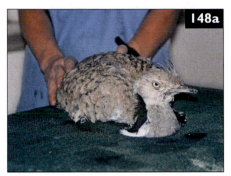 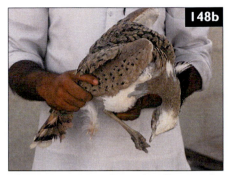

148 An adult Houbara bustard that arrived at a private zoological collection the previous week is presented with a history of inappetence, laboured breathing and a nasal discharge (148a). The bird died overnight and the owner submitted the carcase along with a second live bird from the group, which was showing neurological signs (148b). A further two birds from the original group of eight were head shaking and ataxic. The birds had not been vaccinated.

i. What samples would you collect from the live and the dead bird for laboratory investigation, and how is the diagnosis confirmed?

ii. What are the differential diagnoses for conditions causing upper respiratory signs in bustards?

iii. What recommendations would you make to the manager of this collection to prevent this disease in the future, and are there any risks in maintaining surviving birds in the collection?

149 Rosenberg's goanna (149) is a species native to open forest and woodland in the temperate zones of Australia. Predation by cats and dogs and injuries sustained by motor vehicles are major threats to the species.

i. If an injured specimen is found, can it be legally removed from the wild?

ii. Is this species subject to CITES regulations?

iii. Which item of national legislation governs the import and export of CITES species in Australia?

148 i. Swabs of the nasal discharge, and choanal and tracheal swabs from live birds, should be screened for *Mycoplasma*, *Chlamydophila* and bacterial diseases. Rapid screening tests on faecal samples to rule out avian influenza should be performed. Rapid screening tests on faecal samples to check for paramyxovirus type 1 (PMV-1) should be performed if available. Samples from post-mortem cases include brain, lung, liver, intestine and spleen. Definitive diagnosis of PMV-1 requires virus isolation, demonstration of the viral antigen by immuno-histochemistry or rising specific antibody titres. In unvaccinated birds, positive titres coupled with clinical signs are regarded as strong diagnostic evidence of PMV-1 infection.

ii. Bacterial infections, particularly gram-negative organisms (e.g. *Pseudomonas aeruginosa*, *Proteus mirabilis*, *Escherichia coli*, *Klebsiella* spp.); viral infections (e.g. PMV-1, avian influenza); fungal infection (e.g. *Aspergillus* spp.); infection with *Chlamydophila* spp. and *Mycoplasma* spp.; non-infectious diseases (e.g. nasal plugs, irritation of the upper respiratory tract with dust, toxins or foreign bodies).

iii. Strict quarantine protocols for incoming stock, exclusion of free-living birds and subcutaneous vaccination using commercially available inactivated PMV-1 vaccines for poultry or gamebirds. Live PMV-1 vaccines can be given to bustards by the intranasal and intraocular routes. In other avian species, birds that have survived infection with PMV-1 can become carriers and intermittently shed virus, but this has not been demonstrated in bustards.

149 i. Yes, if removing the animal from the wild will prevent or relieve suffering, the animal may be taken and as a general rule should be transferred to an authorized carer associated with a wildlife rescue organization and licensed by the relevant state government. However, it should be noted that the degree to which various reptile species are protected in the wild varies from state to state.

ii. Yes, all members of the genus *Varanus* are CITES listed.

iii. Part 13A of the Environment Protection and Biodiversity Conservation Act 1999 (EPBC Act). The EPBC Act is the Australian Government's principal piece of environmental legislation and, in addition to regulating the import and export of wildlife and wildlife products, it aims to protect matters of national environmental significance by conserving Australian biodiversity, enhancing the protection and management of important natural and cultural places and by promoting ecologically sustainable development.

150 i. What are the lesions seen on this white-tailed deer (150)?
ii. How is the disease transmitted, and what are the implications for consumption of venison from this animal?

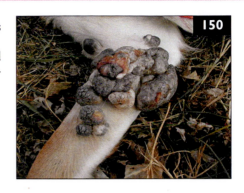

151 i. What species is this (151)?
ii. What is its diet, and how should it be managed in captivity?

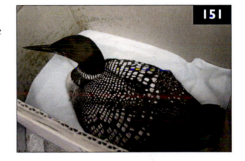

152 An image of the carpal joint of an adult Houbara bustard is shown (152).
i. What does this injury tell you about the possible origins of this bird?
ii. What problems in the birds's environment can lead to this injury?
iii. How can the frequency of such injuries be reduced in centres where birds are being rehabilitated for release into the wild?

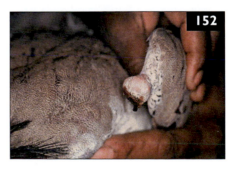

150 i. Cutaneous fibroma. These are hairless tumours, caused by a papillomavirus, found on the skin of white-tailed deer. Clinical problems rarely arise from these masses, but occasionally an animal will develop large growths that will interfere with vision, respiration, feeding and ambulation.

ii. Deer-to-deer transmission is thought to occur through biting insects and possibly also through direct contact with various contaminated materials that may abrade the skin. This is not a zoonotic disease, and only large fibromas with secondary bacterial infection would cause the deer carcase to be unfit for consumption.

151 i. A great northern diver, also known as the common loon in North America.

ii. Small fish. In captivity it should be kept on artificial pools with landing areas. These are heavy birds, so concrete landing areas are not recommended in order to avoid foot lesions. The pools should be large enough that the bird can spend most of its time on the water. Small marine fish can be fed. If frozen fish are used, vitamin supplements (e.g. Fisheater Tablets [Mazuri Zoo Foods]) are essential. Salt tablets should not be needed, as these birds are often found on freshwater lakes as well as in coastal waters. The beak is heavy and sharp and care is needed when handling. Gloves are recommended and the head should always be restrained.

152 i. Injuries like this (and also to the keel) occur when bustards are frightened and fly into the side or roof of enclosures, particularly easily stressed and/or wild-derived individuals.

ii. The size of the enclosure, the availability of hiding areas in the enclosure or the abrasiveness of the material used to form the sides of the enclosure.

iii.

- Using plastic coated foam padding to surround the sides of cages or pens (e.g. in areas where birds are regularly caught such as in hospital or quarantine pens).
- Using shade-cloth or tension netting on the roof and sides of aviaries to cushion the impact resulting from birds flying within a pen.
- Modifying behaviour by taming nervous individuals that are not destined to be released, or housing such birds in naturalistic pens with cover.
- Preventing stress by reducing the number of non-essential people who visit the birds.
- It is thought that Houbara bustards derived from migratory populations may be more restless during the migratory season and more vulnerable to trauma-related deaths.

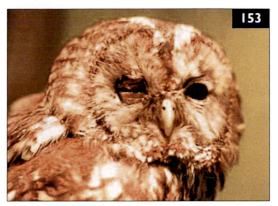

153 An adult tawny owl has been freed from fruit netting after becoming entangled overnight. The bird is in poor body condition and no significant injuries have been found other than a severely damaged right eye (**153**). A clinical examination reveals that the damage to the eye has been present for some time, the globe having partially collapsed.

i. What are the possible courses of action for this bird?

ii. If the bird is kept in captivity as a permanently disabled casualty, what are the welfare implications?

154 The overriding aim of wildlife rehabilitation is the successful release of the casualty back into the wild.

i. Following initial assessment of a wildlife casualty, what are your main options for dealing with it?

ii. What factors would you consider in making your decision?

153 i. The damage to the eye is beyond repair. Enucleation of the entire eyeball in birds, although possible, is difficult due to the size of the globe within the orbit, the reduced orbital musculature and the danger of damage to the contralateral optic nerve during surgery. The options are treatment with suitable antibiotic therapy and monitoring of the condition, surgical 'debulking' of the eyeball, or euthanasia. The bird will inevitably lose the use of one eye and, although many anecdotal reports exist of one-eyed birds surviving in the wild, the ethical position of releasing such a permanently disabled raptor is questionable.

ii. If, after treatment, the injury itself is not causing any concerns regarding welfare, then the possibility is raised of keeping the casualty permanently in captivity. For this the bird should be kept in conditions that are as close to the wild as possible and there should be sound justifications such as: captive breeding programmes for endangered species (not in this case); breeding for legitimate uses (falconry/aviculture); education through licensed use of casualties in conservation presentations; and use in rehabilitation units as imprint models for hand-reared conspecific juveniles).

154 i. The flow chart below shows the main treatment options available:

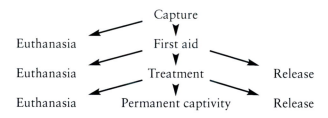

ii. Factors to consider should include: species of casualty and knowledge of its natural history; approximate age of the casualty and, especially, confirmation of whether it is a dependant juvenile or an adult; sex of the casualty; body condition in comparison with what is normal for that species; evidence of acute or chronic problems; heath status, evidence of primary injury or disease; evidence of secondary injuries or disease; psychological status; facilities, knowledge and funding for veterinary treatment and care; facilities, knowledge and funding for rehabilitation and release; likelihood of successful treatment and release in order for the casualty to lead a normal life in the wild, including normal movement, feeding, defence of territory and reproduction; consideration of any negative impacts on wild individuals of the same or another species; availability of suitable release sites.

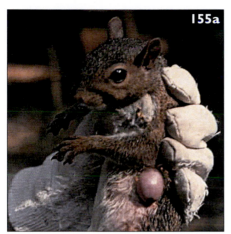

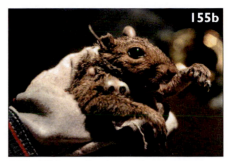

155 This male, juvenile eastern grey squirrel is found with several raised skin lesions (**155a, b**). Each lesion has a circular opening at the apex, and the animal scratches at these intermittently. He is in otherwise good body condition and is demonstrating normal behaviour.

i. What is the cause of the dermal lesions on this squirrel?
ii. How is this condition transmitted, and what species may be affected?
iii. What is the recommended treatment?

156 A juvenile Eurasian sparrowhawk has been found in a garden, close to the house, conscious but unable to fly. On initial examination the bird appears to be in good body condition with no obvious injuries (**156**).

i. If the bird appears to be a suitable candidate for release, what factors should be considered?
ii. If, on initial examination, this bird appeared to be emaciated, how would this affect the approach to the case?

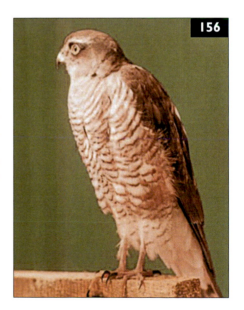

153

155 i. 'Warbles', a bot larva infestation caused by migrating larvae of *Cuterebra emasculator*. Close examination of the lesions reveals a larva within each papule. The opening at the apex of the nodule allows the larva to respire.

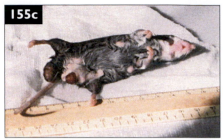

ii. The adult flies lay eggs at burrow entrances, and the larvae gain entrance to the host through the mouth and nostrils. The larvae migrate through the host, eventually entering the subcutis, where they create a hole in the host's skin through which they breathe and excrete waste materials. After approximately three weeks, the full-sized larva drops from the pore and burrows into the soil, where it pupates. Fox squirrels, grey squirrels, woodchucks, cottontail rabbits, mice (155c) and other burrowing or ground-foraging animals (including some birds) have been identified with the larval infestation.

iii. Treatment consists of killing the larvae, careful surgical extraction of the dead larvae and subsequent wound treatment. Larvae may be killed in the skin via topical or oral application of nitenpyram and then removed surgically once dead. Removal of live larvae often leads to an anaphylactic response and death of the affected animal.

156 i. Sparrowhawks frequently collide with windows. It is assumed that, while hunting, they see the movement of their reflection in the glass and, as a reflex, turn towards it as they would towards potential prey. The birds are temporarily stunned and usually recover fully within a short period of time. If presented at a clinic, a short period of detention for observation and stabilization is all that is required. If recovery is not rapid, the possibility of concussion and possible brain damage must be considered, as well as other traumatic injuries (fracture of the coracoid is frequently seen in sparrowhawks, although this presents as obvious wing damage).

All raptors and larger avian casualties (over 500 g) involved in collisions with the risk of head trauma should have, before release, an ophthalmoscopic examination to exclude intraocular haemorrhage caused by impact damage to the pecten.

ii. This may be due to a shortage of food resources or an inability to feed secondary to disease, injury or poor development of feeding skills. Casualties that do not start to feed in captivity or regain body mass are likely to have an inherited or acquired condition that inhibits their survival.

157 A female mallard has some wounds on her dorsal neck and has been anaesthetized using mask induction with isoflurane so that the wounds may be cleaned and dressed (157).

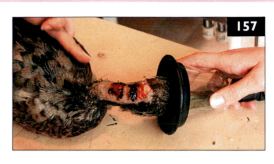

i. What is the likely cause of these wounds?

ii. Does this impact on the release of this bird?

iii. What are the pros and cons associated with this method of anaesthesia in ducks?

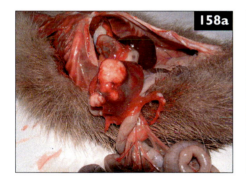

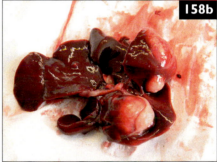

158 This hedgehog presented with severe haemorrhagic vomiting. It was euthanased and post-mortem examination identified large splenic and hepatic abscesses with severe gastritis (158a–c). Enlargement and caseous necrosis of the mesenteric lymph nodes and caseous necrotizing lesions in the Peyer's patches, liver and spleen, typical of this condition, were also found on gross examination.

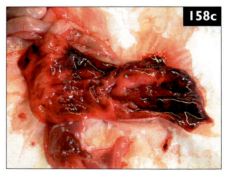

i. What is the cause of this condition?

ii. How is it acquired?

iii. What are the clinical signs?

iv. What is the significance of this condition for wildlife rehabilitators?

157 i. This bird was seen during the mating season and it is most likely that the wounds have been caused by overvigorous mating by one or more male ducks.

ii. The wounds should heal rapidly. However, if the duck is released during the mating season, it is likely that she will be injured again, therefore she should be retained in captivity until after the mating season.

iii. Mask induction of anaesthesia is often rapid and effective in birds. However, ducks may exhibit a 'dive response' with resultant apnoea, meaning that they are very hard to induce and maintain at a surgical plane of anaesthesia. Some veterinary surgeons prefer to induce anaesthesia in waterfowl using injectable agents (e.g. intravenous propofol). The rubber attachment to the mask makes this a semi-open system (rather than fully open). In theory this may be helpful in induction; however, in practice it is unlikely to have any significant effect. The bird can be maintained using an open mask, as this is likely to be a short procedure. Intubation and maintenance on isoflurane given via a T-piece/mechanical ventilation will give better control of the anaesthetic and enable scavenging of waste gases.

158 i. The bacillus *Yersinia pseudotuberculosis*, which is found ubiquitously in the environment.

ii. By ingestion of contaminated food and water, but direct contamination via dust and soil is also possible. The organism can cross the intestinal barrier to reach the underlying Peyer's patches. From there it disseminates to mesenteric lymph nodes, where the bacteria replicate and cause a mesenteric lymphadenitis.

iii. The resulting relatively chronic clinical condition is characterized by weight loss, loss of condition, poor appetite and lethargy. Palpation of the abdomen may identify a number of enlarged lymph nodes. Subacute clinical signs include diarrhoea and weight loss. Affected individuals may die within two weeks to three months. *Y. pseudotuberculosis* can also enter the bloodstream and cause septicaemia, and affected individuals may die within 48 hours. Most cases occur in the winter months. This may be due to the enhanced growth characteristics of the organism in cold temperatures. There is also evidence that transmission is promoted by rodents and migratory birds.

iv. Zoonotic infection may occur in situations where an occupational exposure is likely to arise. Veterinary surgeons and wildlife hospital staff, as well as farmers, hunters and abattoir workers, may be exposed to infected individuals and should therefore take appropriate precautions. Euthanasia of affected wildlife patients is usually recommended due to the zoonotic risk.

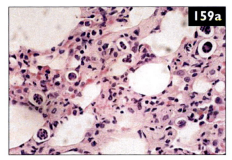

159 You are asked to carry out a post-mortem examination on a red squirrel that was found dead. There is no history. There are no obvious lesions externally or internally, but you submit a range of tissues for histopathological processing. On examination of sections of lung, you observe numerous ovoid multinucleate bodies in the alveolar walls (159a).
i. What are these bodies?
ii. How can you differentiate them from similar structures that might be present in a squirrel's lung?
iii. Are they of clinical significance?

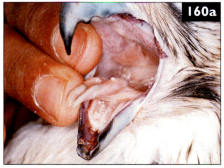
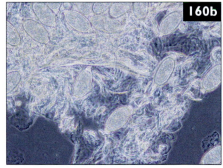

160 A wild peregrine falcon was presented for examination. The bird was underweight and had small yellow plaques present on the oral mucosa (160a). Parasite eggs (160b) were visible when a crop swab was examined.
i. Identify the parasite.
ii. Is infection with this parasite clinically significant?
iii. What is the life cycle of this parasite?
iv. What treatment is recommended?

159 i. Schizonts of the protozoan parasite *Hepatozoon* spp.

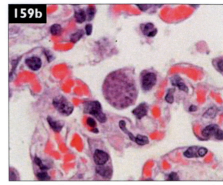

ii. They are most likely to be confused with schizonts of *Toxoplasma gondii*, but are typically larger, oval and have up to 16 dense nuclei. *Toxoplasma* schizonts are less prominent and more variable in form (159b). They are also normally found in other tissues, such as liver and spleen, whereas *Hepatozoon* schizonts are confined to lung.

iii. The significance of *Hepatozoon* infection in red squirrels is currently uncertain, but heavy infections do seem to be associated with alveolar thickening. The species in red squirrels is as yet unnamed, but there is a similar, but genetically distinct, species *Hepatozoon griseisciuri* in grey squirrels.

160 i. *Capillaria* spp. It is easily identified by microscopic examination of faecal samples or mucosal scrapings from lesions in the oropharynx. *Capillaria* eggs are oval and have characteristic bipolar plugs.

ii. Three forms of the disease are recognized in raptors based on the location of the infection: oropharyngeal, oesophageal and intestinal forms. Lesions in the mouth can lead to localized abscesses, oesophageal lesions can rupture through the skin and the intestinal form can result in inflammatory changes causing diarrhoea and weakness.

iii. Earthworms can play a role as transport hosts in the transmission of *Capillaria* to birds of prey. Raptors are also infected with *Capillaria* following ingestion of infected prey.

iv. Treatment can be challenging as the parasite frequently shows multiple drug resistance. Fenbendazole, mebendazole, ivermectin and doramectin have been used. Follow-up faecal samples should be tested to ensure that the parasite has been eliminated.

161 An emaciated adult hare was found dead. There was no evidence of diarrhoeic staining and no palpable impaction in the abdomen. There was staining and matting of the fur around the mouth and on the chin.
i. What are the differential diagnoses?
ii. If this had been a live hare, what particular evaluations should be done prior to consideration for rehabilitation?

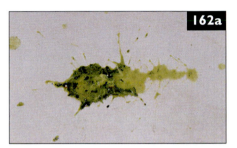

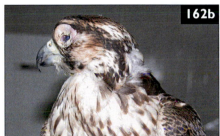

162 A saker falcon was presented for examination with a history of anorexia, biliverdinuria (162a) and a markedly swollen periophthalmic region and infraorbital sinus region (162b). The bird was anaesthetized and radiographed. The lateral radiograph is shown (162c). A blood sample was collected and the significant haematology results included a raised packed cell volume, heterophilia and mono-

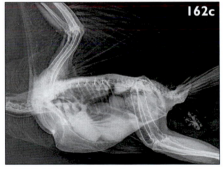

cytosis. A rapid antigen capture test (Speed CHLAM) performed on a swab of the faecal sample for chlamydophilosis was negative.
i. List the conditions that commonly cause these clinical signs in birds?
ii. How reliable is the negative rapid *Chlamydophila* spp. antigen capture test on the faecal sample?
iii. How would you interpret the clinical and laboratory findings, and what further investigative action is indicated?
iv. How would you conclusively confirm your provisional diagnosis?

161 i. Differentials include three conditions causing perioral staining and which have the potential to cause death: (1) leporine dysautonomia, in which impaction is also a major feature; (2) severe dental disease +/- inability to chew and +/- sinus infection; and (3) hare syphilis perioral lesions. In this case there was very severely abnormal cheek tooth development (**161**). A long-

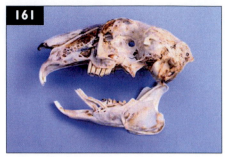

standing infected piercing of a tooth right through the tongue had lead to death from emaciation. Only 2% of hare deaths in one survey were primarily caused by dental disease. In both (2) and (3), death may result from the development of an associated secondary amyloidosis of internal organs (e.g. kidney, liver, spleen or adrenal gland).

ii. A detailed check of the oral cavity, including radiography of the skull.

162 i. Bacterial infection, particularly gram-negative organisms (e.g. *Pseudomonas aeruginosa*), fungal infection (e.g. *Aspergillus* spp.) and infection with *Chlamydophila* spp. Viral infections (e.g. PMV-1, avian influenza) are less common, but should be considered.

ii. Pooled choanal and oropharyngeal swabs are more consistent for isolation of the agent than faecal swabs, especially in the early stages of infection. This bird may have been in the early stages of infection and conducting a rapid antigen test on a faecal sample was not sensitive enough.

iii. The clinical (splenomegaly) and laboratory findings (heterophilia, monocytosis) are suggestive of an infectious disease process, possibly chlamydophilosis. Cytology should be conducted on impression smears of the discharge and samples collected for bacteriology. Examination of paired serum samples to demonstrate rising titres of *Chlamydophila* spp. antibodies should be conducted. Plasma chemistry should be carried out on samples collected before any treatment (including intramuscular injections) is given. This may provide information on hepatic function and hydration status.

iv. Diagnostic methods to confirm *Chlamydophila* spp. infection include:

• Direct visualization in clinical specimens by staining impression smears.
• Isolation of the agent and identification.
• Detection of seroconversion and a fourfold rise in antibody titres, along with clinical signs or pathological findings typical of the disease.
• Detection of antigen (ELISA or PCR).

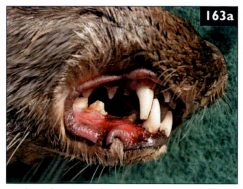

163 You are presented with an adult otter in very weak condition and showing respiratory distress. It has recently lost a lower premolar tooth and the adjacent lip is torn (**163a**).
i. What is the likely cause of these lesions?
ii. What further examinations would you carry out?
iii. Would you attempt treatment, and what is the prognosis?

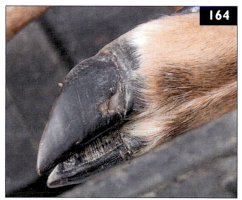

164 **i.** What is the most likely cause of the growth interruption/crack on the hooves of this white-tailed deer (**164**)?
ii. Describe the other clinical and gross pathological signs seen in deer with this disease.

163 i. A fight with another otter. It is very likely that there will be further bite wounds around the face, on the feet and lower limbs and around the perineum.

ii. Although desirable, further examination would be unwise unless the animal can be sedated or anaesthetized, as even sick otters can inflict severe bite wounds. The fact that this otter is showing respiratory distress is a complication, as it is likely to be suffering from pleurisy and/or heart lesions. Purulent pleurisy and pericarditis in an otter resulting from an infected tooth is shown (**163b**). These are common sequelae in otters with infected bite wounds or fractured teeth. As a result they carry a high anaesthetic risk.

iii. A broad-spectrum antibiotic can be given by injection initially, restraining the otter with a grasper. If its condition improves, further examinations while sedated may be justified. However, the prognosis is grave.

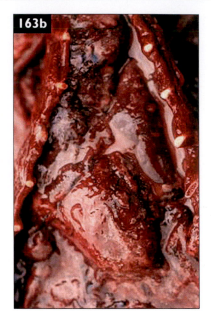

164 i. Chronic haemorrhagic disease caused by epizootic haemorrhagic disease virus or bluetongue virus, which are related, but genetically distinct, *Orbivirus* species. Transmission occurs through biting *Culicoides* midges.

ii. Clinical signs are highly variable. Many deer show no, or only mild, clinical signs, or it can present as a peracute, acute or chronic disease. Initially, animals may exhibit depression, fever, respiratory distress, oedema of the head, neck, conjunctiva or tongue, and cyanosis of the oral mucosa. Deer will typically be found close to a water source. Some animals will die shortly after the onset of clinical signs, but some will live longer and display lameness, inappetence and reduced activity. Gross pathological lesions will also vary depending on the virulence of the virus and duration of infection. Peracute cases will have severe oedema of the head, neck, conjunctiva and lungs. In the acute form the animal will also have petechial haemorrhages in the heart, pulmonary artery, lungs, rumen and intestines. There may also be areas of necrosis or ulcerations on the dental pad, tongue, hard palate, rumen and omasum. The chronic form is typified by hoof growth interruptions as well as sloughing of the hoof walls, and scarring, with loss of papillae, on the rumen mucosa.

165 An emaciated juvenile hedgehog dies within a few hours of being found out during the daytime. On necropsy, the mesentery contains multiple haemorrhages and there are approximately 50 small cream-coloured, seed-like structures approximately 5 mm in length throughout (**165a**).

i. What are these structures?

ii. How could their identification be confirmed?

iii. Could they be responsible for the death of this hedgehog?

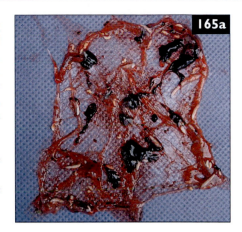

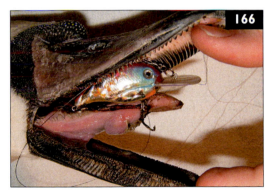

166 A mute swan (**166**) from a local lake is presented to your practice by members of a local wildlife charity.

i. What type of fishing gear is pictured here, and what special problems can this cause?

ii. How would you remove this item and treat the swan?

iii. Would you carry out any diagnostic procedures in this case?

165 i. Thorny-headed worms (Acanthocephala).
ii. Direct microscopy of the cranial portion of the worm will show the characteristic hooks (165b).
iii. Yes. Although usually found in small numbers and of little significance in hedgehogs, occasionally, extreme cases with large numbers of worms are encountered with widespread intestinal ulceration, haemorrhage and anaemia, which can prove fatal. There may, however, be an underlying disorder causing immunosuppression predisposing to such a large Acanthocephala burden. The most commonly found species are *Moniliformis erinacei* and *Prosthorhyncus* spp.

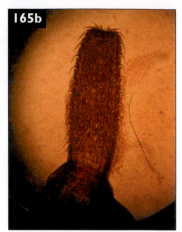

166 i. A triple-barbed pike hook. This can cause severe damage to the tongue and bill. One hook penetrates the tongue, one penetrates or damages the bill and the other remains pointing out, which can make it difficult and dangerous to the person removing it. The associated line is usually reinforced and may cause substantial trauma if it wraps around the bill.
ii. It is easier, safer and less stressful to remove the hook under anaesthesia or sedation. Free points should be cut off using wirecutters, wearing eye protection and holding the tips in forceps to avoid injury. Any points entering tissue should be cut at the base and drawn out in the direction of the barbs to avoid further tissue damage. Simple penetrative damage is usually minor, but ligation of the tongue by line or repeated excoriation by a free hook point can cause distal tongue necrosis. Local cleaning and débridement are advised, together with parenteral antibiosis and analgesia. Fluid therapy and nutritional support are advisable. The tongue usually heals rapidly, but any distal tissue necrosis results in a poor prognosis if the bird cannot feed for itself.
iii. Survey radiographs are advised to check for internal hooks, line and weights and any other hooks that may be embedded in wing webs or feet.

167 What is the significance of psittacine beak and feather disease (PBFD) to wild psittacine populations in Australia?

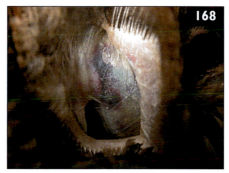

168 The ear of a tawny owl is shown (**168**).
i. What lesion can be seen?
ii. What is the significance of this?

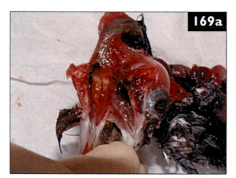

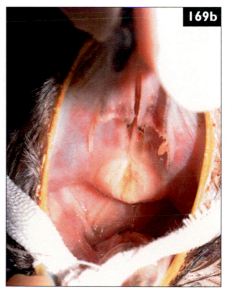

169 i. What is the likely cause of the lesions visible on the post-mortem examinations in this chaffinch (**169a**) and buzzard (**169b**)?
ii. How does the epidemiology of this condition differ between birds of prey, finches and pigeons?

167 PBFD is endemic at high prevalence in wild lorikeet flocks, so eradicating the disease from wild populations is not feasible. PBFD was listed in April 2001 as a key threatening process to endangered Australian psittacines (Australian Environment Protection and Biodiversity Conservation Act 1999). Artificial congregation of large numbers of birds at feeders probably aids in the transmission of the virus. Evidence suggests that recovered lorikeets remain latently infected, with the virus persisting in their livers. Releasing rehabilitated recovered birds can be problematic, as it increases the general viral load in wild populations and could affect sympatric populations of endangered psittacine species.

168 i. There is bruising evident overlying the bone enclosing the globe.
ii. There is likely to have been cranial trauma and, as the bone is so thin, almost certainly haemorrhage from the pecten of the eye into the posterior chamber (even if no haemorrhage can be seen in the anterior chamber). It is essential that this bird receives a full ocular examination. It can be difficult to achieve mydriasis in order to examine the posterior chamber. The easiest way is to anaesthetize the bird. If there is haemorrhage present, then topical anti-inflammatories (e.g. corticosteroids) should be used. Resolution of the haemorrhage should be monitored and if retinal detachment results, then the bird is not a candidate for release.

169 i. Infection with the protozoal parasite *Trichomonas gallinae*.
ii. *T. gallinae* is a cosmopolitan parasite of pigeons and doves and is readily transmitted to squabs through the feeding of crop milk. The organism thus cycles from one generation of pigeons to another. In addition to the direct form of transmission from parent birds to young seen in pigeons, two additional modes of transmission may occur.

Birds of prey, such as buzzards, prey on wood pigeons and may become infected with the parasite when feeding on infected material. The incidence of trichomonosis in other birds of prey known to feed on pigeons (e.g. Eurasian sparrowhawks and peregrine falcons), does not appear to be as great as that in the more opportunistic buzzard. Garden bird trichomonosis is now recognized as an emerging disease of wild greenfinches, chaffinches and goldfinches.

The epidemiology underpinning the emergence of this new form of the disease has not been elucidated. It is, however, likely that it involves the contamination of feeding and drinking stations. The trichomonad organism does not survive for long outside of the host, but water-borne transmission is likely where large numbers of birds are encouraged to congregate and heavy contamination of a water bath or bird table is allowed.

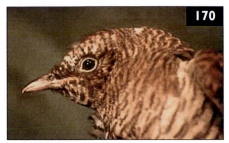

170 In late summer, a juvenile common cuckoo (170) is presented having been found in a rural garden. The bird is in fair body condition and on examination the only injury that can be found is a fracture of the right tarsometatarsus. The bird responds well to hand feeding. What considerations are important in the assessment of this case?

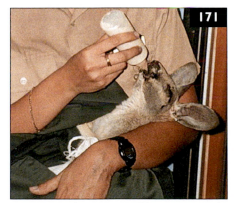

171 A carer hand rearing an orphan joey red kangaroo is shown (171). Diarrhoea is one of the most common presenting complaints in such animals. List the causes of diarrhoea in hand-raised macropods.

172 A group of badger cubs has been hand reared. A suitable release site has been found and landowner consent for the release has been gained. The farmer is concerned about the risk of *M. bovis* infection to his cattle on the adjacent land.
i. How would you go about testing this group of animals for tuberculosis?
ii. What are the disadvantages associated with testing?

170 This case highlights the importance of knowledge of the natural history of an individual undergoing rehabilitation. Hand rearing an insectivorous juvenile should present few problems and in passerine birds, fractures to a tarsometatarsal bone usually heal without complications when immobilized externally by splinting. However, cuckoos are migrants and this fracture will take several weeks to heal. By late summer most juvenile cuckoos are independent of their foster parents and about to start their southward migration. This bird will not be fit for release for at least 3–4 weeks, which means that it will have to start its migration immediately and, although the autumn migration is usually taken in short stages, this bird will not be in a fit state to perform long periods of exertion. A decision will have to be made on the ethics of releasing a bird unlikely to be fit enough to embark on migration, of retaining the bird in captivity over the winter or, on humane grounds, of performing euthanasia.

171 Causes of diarrhoea are usually multifactorial in hand-reared joeys, but are often related to suboptimal husbandry. In general, the more consistent and standardized the husbandry routine the better. Possible causes of diarrhoea in hand-reared joeys include: oral and intestinal candidiasis (secondary to stress, immuno-suppression, poor husbandry); lactose intolerance (incorrect rearing formula); malabsorption (excessive volume or secondary to bacterial overgrowth); bacterial diarrhoea (secondary to inadequate hygiene or inappropriate administration of antibiotics); coccidiosis (only seen in recently pouch emerged grazing joeys, especially eastern greys); helminths (rare until animal is grazing); psychological diarrhoea (secondary to stress associated with poor management).

172 **i.** The methods of testing individual badgers for tuberculosis all have their limitations. None of the current methods of testing have a high enough sensitivity to ensure individual animals are free from infection. The badger Tb ELISA test was developed for use in groups of animals and would be an appropriate test to detect infection on a group basis, but not to indicate infection in individual animals, as its sensitivity is too low (40.7%). In individual animals the sensitivity of the Tb ELISA can be increased to acceptable levels (over 80%) by using three applications of the test. The time badger cubs spend in captivity allows for the use of multiple testing, usually at admission, weaning and before release.
ii. Multiple testing increases the sensitivity of the badger Tb ELISA, but at some cost to its specificity (reduced from 94.3% to 83.1%). Badgers may therefore test ELISA positive, but be negative on standard post-mortem examination and culture tests following euthanasia. Other disadvantages include the necessity to sedate or anaesthetize all but the very smallest cubs in order to collect blood safely. The cost of testing three times may also be prohibitive in some situations.

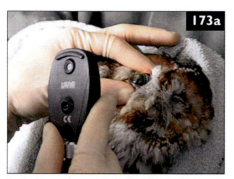

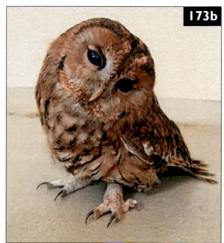

173 Complete ophthalmological examination (173a) is a crucial part of any clinical examination in injured birds and should not be overlooked.
i. Why is this?
ii. Why might it be of particular importance in birds of prey such as this tawny owl (173b)?

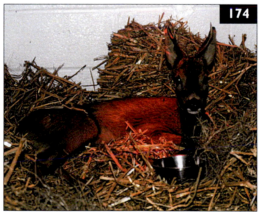

174 A roe deer (174) has been captured and held overnight in captivity. How would you anaesthetize this animal in order to suture a wound on its flank?

173 i. Ophthalmological examination is vital in the assessment of casualty wild birds undergoing rehabilitation back to the wild, as a visual deficit may prevent a bird from finding and killing sufficient prey to sustain itself. Prey species are particularly reliant on their vision to avoid predators.

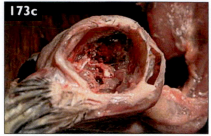

ii. Visual impairment in an owl may affect its ability to avoid obstacles and may even prevent it from flying. Many lesions affect the posterior segment and would be missed if a complete ophthalmological examination is not performed. In raptors the eyes constitute a major portion of the cranial mass and they are particularly vulnerable to trauma. This tawny owl presented with a head tilt and central blindness. The large size of the owl's orbit and the absence of a prominent supraorbital ridge make it vulnerable to trauma. Haemorrhaging within the retrobulbar tissues can be seen adjacent to the optic nerve (**173c**).

Significant ophthalmological lesions were found in 75% of 128 wild tawny owls presented to a UK wildlife hospital. This study also found that the Schirmer tear test was consistently lower than found in some other families of birds. This may increase pathology of the cornea in tawny owls and should be considered when deciding on treatment protocols.

174 Deer are both difficult to handle and easily stressed by handling procedures. Intramuscular injections may be used as the sole anaesthetic agents for short procedures. A combination of ketamine (2–3 mg/kg) plus an alpha-2 adrenergic agonist, such as xylazine (2 mg/kg) or medetomidine (50–100 µg/kg), is most appropriate. Medetomidine has the advantage that it can be reversed using atipamazole (200 µg/kg). Both sedative combinations, together with local anaesthesia (procaine or lidocaine), are suitable for suturing of small wounds.

Intravenous lines placed to prevent 'shock' and capture myopathy allow for intravenous induction of anaesthesia with minimal handling. Premedication with diazepam (0.5 mg/kg i/v) reduces the amount of induction agent required and aids intubation. Ketamine (3 mg/kg i/v) can be used for induction following premedication with xylazine (2 mg/kg i/v). Alternatively, propofol (2–4 mg/kg i/v slowly to effect) may be used. It can also be used to maintain field anaesthesia as a bolus (0.6–1.5 mg/kg) or continuous infusion. Isoflurane or sevoflurane in oxygen can be used to maintain anaesthesia following sedation or induction. Deer are relatively easily intubated using suitably sized (8–12 mm for adult roe deer) cuffed endotracheal tubes.

Recovery following general anaesthesia should be in a quiet, darkened and, ideally, padded recovery box.

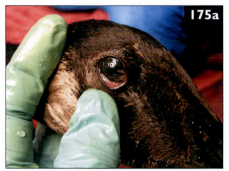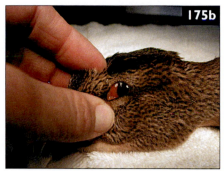

175 Some unusual ocular lesions are noted during a routine examination of a Canada goose captured in an oil spill (**175a**). Similar lesions have also been found in a chuck-will's-widow, a mallard (**175b**) and several species of gull.

i. What is the aetiology of this condition?

ii. How should this condition be treated?

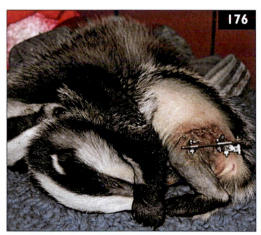

176 **i.** What does this image show (**176**)?

ii. What makes both this individual and the method of fixation used advantageous to a successful outcome?

175 i. These birds have flukes (*Philophthalmus gral*) embedded in the conjunctiva deep to the nictitating membrane. The birds ingest encysted cercariae on an intermediate aquatic host, such as a snail or crayfish. The flukes migrate through the avian gastrointestinal tract to the ocular mucosa.

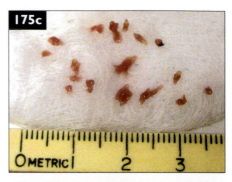

ii. The affected bird can be anaesthetized and the flukes manually removed using eye dressing forceps (175c, d). The application of ophthalmic tetracaine drops (0.5%) five minutes prior to the procedure results in easier removal of the flukes and less inflammation afterwards. Topical ophthalmic lubricants alone or combined with a topical ophthalmic anti-inflammatory for 1–2 days afterwards may also help to alleviate discomfort and decrease healing time.

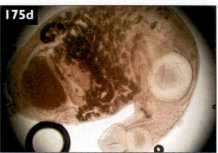

176 i. A badger cub (approximately eight weeks old) with an external skeletal fixator system applied to a femoral fracture of its left hindlimb. The system is made up of an intramedullary pin 'tied-in' to a unilateral, uniplantar half frame (lateral supporting bar with angulated positive profile pins), which maintains alignment and stability at the fracture site and prevents rotation.

ii. Because this injury has occurred in a cub, the fracture should heal quickly (4–6 weeks maximum). A badger cub would normally be kept in captivity for several months before release, so fracture healing is unlikely to delay its release. In adult mammals the time in captivity required for fractures to heal may limit the likelihood of the casualty being successfully released because of complications associated with long-term captivity.

The metal implants (pin and external system) are removed once the fracture is healed, allowing the casualty to be released without possible future complications of implants being left in place. If plates, screws and cerclage wires are used to stabilize fractures, they should also be removed if possible, though this is often much more difficult. Screws, pins and wires may work loose over a period of time, causing local reaction and leading to osteomyelitis. Retained implants should be avoided wherever possible in wildlife casualties.

177 i. What species of bird is this (177a)?

ii. What are the lesions on the legs likely to be caused by?

iii. What pathogens are also reported to be associated with these lesions?

iv. What treatment options, if any, are available in this case?

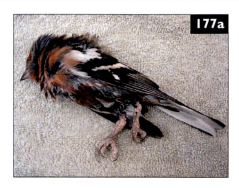

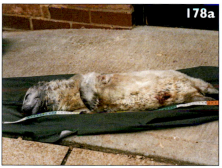

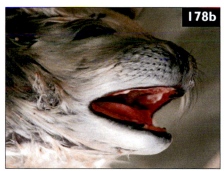

178 This seal (178a, b) was found alive on the beach in eastern England in mid-May. The animal was in respiratory distress and died while being transported to a rehabilitation centre.

i. What species is this seal, and what can you say from its external appearance?

ii. Suggest a probable cause for the respiratory distress and death?

iii. How could this be confirmed?

179 What criteria should be considered when selecting the best time and place to release orphan cygnets?

177 i. A chaffinch.
ii. Mites (*Cnemidocoptes* spp.) (**177b**).
iii. Viral papillomas have been shown to occur in clusters in finches, especially chaffinches. Studies show a prevalence of 1.3%. On histopathology a hyper-keratotic epidermis with intranuclear inclusion bodies may be seen.
iv. Topical application of ivermectin or fipronil. There is no treatment for papillomas and often these birds require euthanasia.

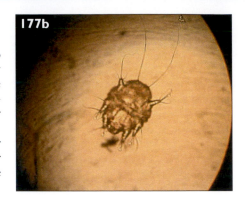

178 i. A harbour seal. It has a 'step' in its forehead and a triangular rhinarium typical of the species. In the UK, the harbour seal pupping season is June and July. Harbour seals have a white lanugo coat, like other true seals (the grey seal and ice breeding seals such as harp and ringed seals), but unlike other species they lose this lanugo coat before birth. Harbour seals resemble adults phenotypically at birth and the shed lanugo coat can be found in the birth fluids. Seals have permanent teeth erupted at birth and do not have a temporary dentition.
ii. This seal has a lanugo coat and a fresh, bloody umbilical stump. The teeth have not yet erupted. This is a case of premature birth. Respiratory distress and death may well be connected with incomplete lung inflation due to prematurity.
iii. This could be confirmed by evidence of poorly inflated lungs on necropsy. The timing of this stranding (mid-May, before the start of the breeding season in this region) is consistent with this conclusion. Pacific harbour seals are frequently seen at birth in lanugo coat, which they lose within a few days. This is a normal variation in this subspecies.

179 Ideally, they should be reared with other orphan cygnets and released when they have attained their full plumage (i.e. their flight feathers), which in the case of mute swans is September to the end of November in the northern hemisphere. They should be released where there is a group of wintering swans that are support fed. This can be a river estuary or other water body. The support feeding will help them through their first winter before they decide to disperse.

180 You are presented with an American mink, which was killed by a gamekeeper in Somerset, UK. It is in good condition and the liver appears normal, but the gallbladder is thick walled and pink and there are numerous blackish bodies, less than 1 mm long, on the mucosal surface (**180a**).

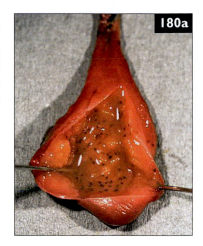

i. What is your provisional diagnosis?
ii. How would you confirm it?
iii. What other species may be infected?

181 i. What species is this (**181**)?
ii. What is its natural diet?
iii. What factors should be considered prior to its release back into the wild following a period of rehabilitation?

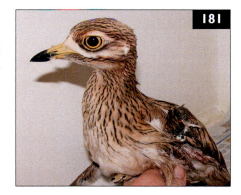

182 This pipistrelle bat (**182**) was found alive on someone's garden path. It was submitted to a bat hospital and ate well for two days and appeared to be recovering. On the third day it stopped eating and died.

i. What is likely to have caused the damage to the wing membrane?
ii. What is the probable cause of death?

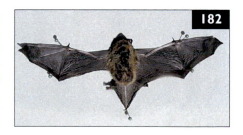

180 i. Cholecystitis, caused by the bile fluke *Pseudamphistomum truncatum*.

ii. By transferring several of the small bodies to a microscope slide, adding a small amount of water and examining them with a compound microscope using a low-power objective and a lowered condenser. *P. truncatum* from the gallbladder of a mink are shown (180b).

iii. *P. truncatum* is commonly found in UK otters in Somerset and Dorset and in East Anglia. In Europe the parasite has also been recorded in a wide range of carnivores, including foxes, polecats and domestic cats and dogs. There are rare reports of infection in humans. The life cycle involves freshwater crustaceans and certain species of fish. Infection can only be acquired by eating uncooked fish.

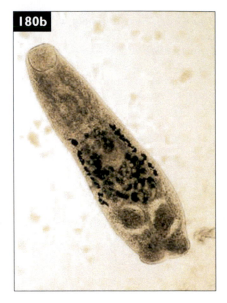
180b

181 i. A stone curlew, also known as the Eurasian thick-knee.

ii. Leafy plants and invertebrates, which are easily provided in captivity.

iii. It is a shy bird and is largely crepuscular or nocturnal. Therefore, in captivity, brightly lit areas should be avoided and the bird should be given as much seclusion as possible. In some areas of the UK this species is the subject of conservation work and monitoring. Areas of pasture are often managed as 'stone curlew plots'. If planning to release such a bird, it is important to liaise with local groups to ensure release into the correct area and, of course, enable post-release monitoring.

182 i. Bites from a domestic cat.

ii. In such cases there are often other internal injuries not readily detected on clinical examination. These include torn pectoral muscles, ruptured abdominal wall and ruptured liver. However, if the bat initially improves and then dies after approximately 48–72 hours, it is usually due to *Pasteurella* septicaemia. *P. multocida* is a commensal in cats' mouths and is introduced via bite wounds. In rehabilitation centres it is a common cause of death in birds as well as in bats and other small mammals.

183 An immature mute swan is presented (**183**). The bird has been present on a local river for several days, with a very obviously damaged wing. It has been the cause of much public concern and has eventually been captured in a widely publicized rescue. On examination the bird appears to be in poor body condition. No other injuries are found other than an open, comminuted fracture

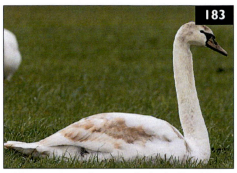

of the distal third of the right humerus, with a section of exposed, devitalized bone and infection of the associated soft tissue. The public interest in this case has resulted in many offers of financial assistance and sites for relocating the bird. What are the options for dealing with this injury?

184 A young passerine bird is presented with weakness and masses over the head (**184**).
i. What is the likely cause?
ii. How would you manage this case?

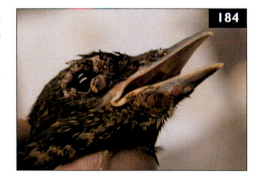

185 i. What are the likely causes of the injury in this hedgehog (**185**)?
ii. What would be your medical considerations in treating this case?

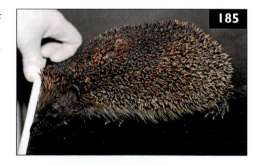

183 Such injuries are commonly the result of mid-air collisions with power cables and by the time the bird is captured the injuries, as in this case, have probably gone beyond surgical repair. Amputation or euthanasia are the only options. The release of a wing amputee into the wild is clearly unethical. However, the possibility does exist to release such a casualty onto a small, privately owned stretch of water that is not the territory of an existing pair of breeding swans, but this situation would need constant supervision to ensure the welfare of the casualty. Such cases are often exposed to the full glare of publicity and they highlight the necessity of educating the public in the realities of dealing with wildlife casualties.

184 i. Avipox infection. There is heavy crusting with secondary infection on the eyelids and this is likely to cause scarring. If scarring is severe, there may be permanent damage to the eyelids and cornea.
ii. There is no specific therapy; however, if secondary bacterial infections can be controlled and the bird is provided with appropriate supportive care and can self-feed, it is likely to resolve in a few weeks. Avipoxvirus is spread both by insect vectors and by direct contact, gaining entry to the skin via open wounds. Therefore, good barrier nursing and fly control are essential if this bird is to be admitted and nursed in a wildlife hospital.

185 i. The hedgehog is showing generalized blackening and shortening of the cranial dorsal spines consistent with burn injuries. Hedgehogs frequently nest in piles of leaves and wood prepared as bonfires and become injured in this way when the fires are lit.
ii. A full clinical examination should be performed to assess the severity of burning as well as to look for any concurrent disease or injury. The spines may become fused when burnt and this may compromise the ability of the animal to roll. Skin damage below the spines may not become evident for several days, after which the skin begins to slough. Burnt hedgehogs should be kept in captivity and closely observed for at least one week to ensure there are no such delayed problems. Topical treatment of damaged skin is often difficult, but cleaning of affected areas with sterile saline or a dilute solution of chlorhexidine, followed by the application of a cream containing silver sulfadiazine or cleansing agents, may be beneficial. Broad-spectrum anti-bacterials (e.g. potentiated amoxicillin) given orally are indicated where skin damage is marked. Lung damage through smoke inhalation is an additional complication requiring oxygen therapy in the early stages of treatment, together with the use of anti-inflammatory drugs, bronchodilators and broad-spectrum antibacterials.

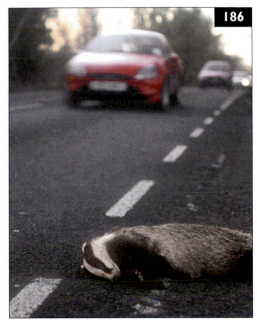

186 Land mammals are frequently involved in road traffic accidents (RTAs) (**186**).
i. What are the common injuries sustained?
ii. How would you deal with RTAs, and what prognosis would you attach to the various types of injury?

187 i. How can dehydration be assessed in wild birds?
ii. By what routes can fluids be administered?

186 i. Fractures of long bones and/or pelvis; lung contusions, pneumothorax, haemothorax; diaphragm rupture; liver or spleen contusions and/or rupture; bladder rupture; damage to the central nervous system; brain injuries, spinal injuries, peripheral nerve damage.

ii. As with all wildlife casualties, the normal 'triage' considerations must be made. These include the general condition of the casualty and presence of concurrent disease or injury, species-specific considerations related to its ability to return to full normal function and consideration of rehabilitation facilities and release sites. All cases are likely to require immediate first aid treatment, usually including fluid therapy (colloids or crystalloids) and analgesia (NSAID and opioid drugs), and the provision of a warm environment to prevent further heat loss and slowly return body temperature to normal. Diagnostic tests include radiography, ultrasonography of the thorax and abdomen, diagnostic abdominocentesis and thoracocentesis, exploratory laparotomy and blood tests to assess the haematological and biochemical status.

Some injuries may resolve with supportive treatment (e.g. contusions to lung, liver or spleen, inflammatory CNS damage, mild pneumothorax or haemothorax). Surgical treatment of some injuries carries a good prognosis (e.g. splenectomy, diaphragm repair) and others a reasonable prognosis (e.g. liver lobectomy, fracture repair). The surgical skills of the veterinary surgeon, facilities and funding available must be considered.

187 i. The high metabolic rate of birds results in rapid fluid deficits after a short period of anorexia. Avian skin is much thinner and less pliable than mammalian skin, making assessment of skin tenting more difficult. Dehydration status can be assessed as follows: <5%, imperceptible signs; 5–6%, loss of skin elasticity, skin slides less readily over breast muscles; 7–10%, skin dry and adherent, buccal mucosa dry with presence of false membranes in the mouth, cornea dull; 10–12%, generalized weakness/collapse, changes in scale colour on legs and feet (dull beige instead of bright yellow), cold extremities, cornea dry; >12%, extreme weakness/collapse.

ii. All wild avian casualties should be considered at least 5% dehydrated and receive oral fluids (2.5% body weight) as part of initial first aid. If too sick or stressed to receive oral fluids, an intraosseous or intravenous catheter can be placed, which may require anaesthesia. Intraosseous catheters should be placed in non-pneumatized bones, such as the proximal tibiotarsus and the distal and proximal ulna, and they can be capped and protected with a suitably shaped finger splint, applied over a figure of eight bandage. Boluses of fluid can be administered at regular intervals, or via a giving set to large birds. Suitable vessels for intravenous catheter placement include the ulnar, basilic, medial metatarsal and saphenous veins.

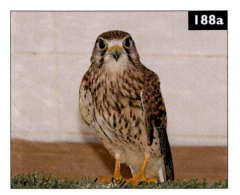

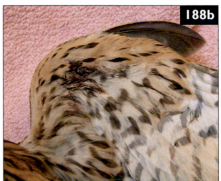

188 i. What species is shown (**188a**)?
Can you give an idea of its sex or age?
ii. What lesions can be seen (**188b, c**)?
iii. How can this be managed?

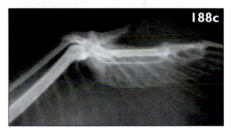

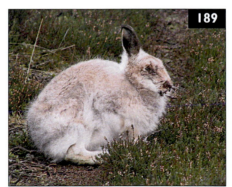

189 i. What is this species (**189**)?
ii. What clinical signs can you see from the photo?
iii. What are your differential diagnoses?
iv. How would you treat this case?

188 i. A common kestrel. The brown head, wing tips and tail show that this is either an immature bird or an adult female. The adult male has a slate grey head, tail and wing tips.

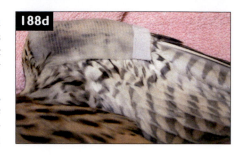

ii. The distal left wing is drooping, indicating injury to (or just distal to) the carpus. A wound is visible in the metacarpal region. The radiograph shows a fracture of the metacarpal bones.

iii. There is little bone displacement; however, the fracture is complicated by being open. Systemic antibiosis and NSAIDs are indicated. This type of fracture will not heal without support. In this case a piece of thermoplastic was shaped and moulded to the ventral distal wing (188d) so that it bent upwards over the edge of the wing. This was held in place with tape for five days. If the dressing is in place for longer than five days, there is likely to be muscle and joint contracture. If the fracture is not healed at this time, the dressing should be left off for two days before being reapplied for five more days. If still not healed, the fracture should be reinvestigated to determine the cause of the non-union.

189 i. Blue hare (syn. mountain hare, Arctic hare, Irish hare, varying hare). It is distinguishable from the brown hare by its smaller size, shorter ears and greyer coat, which in winter becomes white with dark ear tips. This picture was taken in early December with the coat in transitional pelage. It is found in Ireland and the Scottish Highlands, especially on managed heather grouse moors.
ii. Crusting lesions around the nose, lips and eyelids.
iii. Myxomatosis, pasteurellosis, treponematosis.
iv. Wild hare are difficult to capture and keep in captivity and treatment is therefore difficult. Clinical myxomatosis carries a poor prognosis, with no treatment for the primary viral cause. Pasteurellosis may be treated with antibacterials, but permanent respiratory tract damage may result and recurrence of clinical disease is not uncommon. Treponematosis can be treated with parenteral penicillin (40 mg/kg q24h for 5 days).

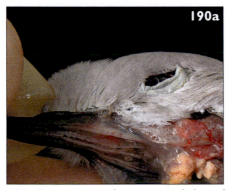 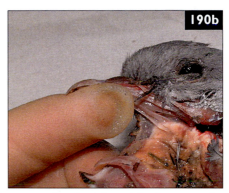

190 Dyspnoea and open mouth breathing, associated with weight loss, may be seen in pigeons and doves.
i. What is the likely cause of these clinical signs and the post-mortem lesions shown in these doves (190a, b)?
ii. How can the diagnosis be confirmed?

191 i. What does this radiograph show (191)?
ii. How would you treat this fracture in this wild animal, and what would affect your decision making in this case?

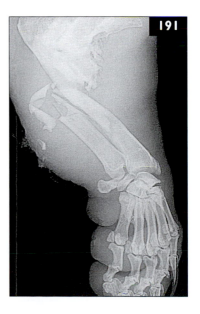

190 i. The flagellated protozoal parasite *Trichomonas gallinae* is responsible for the oropharyngeal lesions shown here in a collared dove (**190a**) and a stock dove (**190b**). As many as 80% of pigeons are silent carriers of this organism. Pathogenic strains of the organism are able to take advantage of small lesions in the oropharyngeal mucosa. Rapid multiplication leads to extensive ulceration and the formation of caseous material that

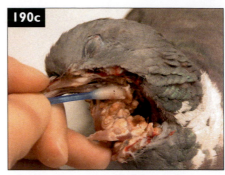

190c

can cause obstruction of the respiratory and digestive tracts. Build up of caseous material around the choanae and glottis can give rise to considerable respiratory difficulty. Trichomonosis is becoming increasingly recognized as a cause of disease and increased mortality in wild pigeons and doves.
ii. By identification of motile protozoa in oropharyngeal swab material. Samples should be taken from live birds or 'still warm' cadavers in order to maximize the likelihood of detecting motility. This is done by collecting a sample using a saline moistened cotton swab (**190c**) and expressing a drop of fluid onto a microscope slide. Culture of the organism from swabs placed in an appropriate transport medium is also possible.

191 i. A mid-shaft, compound comminuted fracture of the radius and ulna of a large mammal, in this case a badger (the five full digits suggest it is not a canid). There is abnormal bone proliferation around the elbow joint, most notably on the cranial aspect of the distal humerus and proximal radius. This suggests the fracture is associated with chronic disease. It is likely that the bone had become weakened at the fracture site as a result of the changes proximal to it. The new bone formation might be due to osteomyelitis resulting from a bite wound or other penetrating infection. Neoplasia is a possible but less likely cause.
ii. Fracture fixation, amputation of the limb or euthanasia. Fracture fixation is likely to carry a poor prognosis, as the fracture site includes diseased bone. Fracture healing is likely to be poor and the elbow joint will remain compromised. As this is an adult animal (all growth plates appear closed on the radiograph), the time in captivity would be protracted. The need to remove any orthopaedic metal implants prior to release also limits the methods of possible fixation. As this is a large mammal requiring forelimbs for both normal locomotion and digging, amputation is not an ethical course of action. Euthanasia would be the author's preferred option in this case.

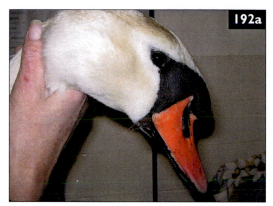

192 A mute swan was reported by a member of the general public 48 hours ago as appearing distressed. The swan has now been captured and is presented to you. How would you deal with this casualty based on the photo shown (**192a**)?

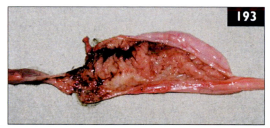

193 A small otter cub was found in weak condition, apparently abandoned. It was taken into care and improved for a few days, but then developed blackish diarrhoea and died. On post-mortem examination the stomach was empty apart from blackish deposits over the mucosa in the pyloric region, and the mucosa itself was ulcerated (**193**). The intestines contained blackish mucoid material. Bacterial cultures of stomach and intestines failed to demonstrate any pathogens.
i. What is the blackish material over the pyloric mucosa?
ii. What is the likely cause of the lesions?

192 The image shows fishing line at the swan's bill. Fishing line and hook injuries are common in swans. Fluid therapy should be administered to stabilize the casualty prior to anaesthesia, especially where there has been a known delay in capture. Anaesthesia is required for full assessment and removal of most hooks and lines. Gaseous agents (isoflurane or sevoflurane) may be used for induction via a mask, or intravenous agents (propofol or alfaxalone) can be used. Where hooks and line are limited to the bill, these may be easily removed. Barbed hooks sometimes need to be advanced and cut to allow removal. Where the hook is not visible and line extends down the oesophagus, radiography or endoscopy is essential for assessing the hook position (**192b**). Line must never just

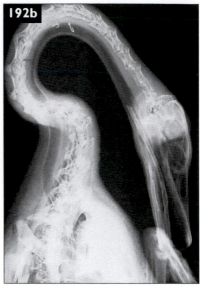

192b

be pulled, as this can cause severe oesophageal damage. Hooks in the oesophagus and proventriculus require removal, while those in the gizzard are rapidly broken down by normal gizzard action and can be left *in situ*. Palpation of the oesophagus may indicate areas of obstruction. Hooks in the oesophagus with line attached can be dislodged using a plastic tube passed over the line to move the hook caudally. Alternatively, hooks can be removed endoscopically or via a surgical incision.

193 i. Changed blood that has escaped from the ulcers. This, together with bile and mucus, forms the bulk of the material in the intestines.
ii. The condition is not due to an infectious agent, but is believed to be a result of stress. Cubs in these situations typically have enlarged adrenal glands. Ulceration of the pyloric mucosa is commonly seen in cubs that are being hand reared, especially by inexperienced people.

194   Badgers (**194a**) may become infected with *Mycobacterium bovis* (bovine tuberculosis).
i. What are the clinical signs associated with this disease in badgers?
ii. What are the options for testing badgers for *M. bovis* infection?

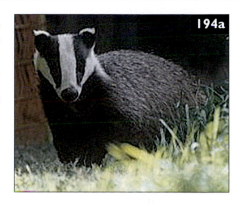

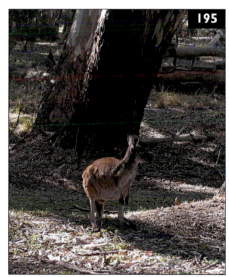

195 i. List four drug combinations that would be suitable for inducing general anaesthesia in this free-ranging western grey kangaroo (**195**).
ii. How should these drugs be administered?
iii. What condition is likely to result from a prolonged chase prior to drug administration in this species?

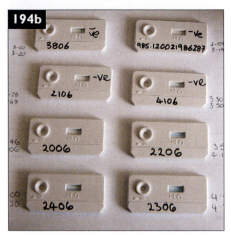

194 i. Some animals may show no or few clinical signs, with infection becoming latent or even resolving. Clinically infected animals show weight loss. There may be an increased likelihood of intraspecies aggression due to the debilitation leading to wounding, which may be a source of *M. bovis* infection. Peripheral lymphadenopathy may be associated with respiratory lesions and wounding. Clinical signs associated with the site of infection may also be evident, lung lesions being most common followed by those in the kidney and GI tract.

ii. Clinical sampling (culture of sputum, faeces, urine and bite wound swabs). The sensitivity of such tests is relatively poor and the time taken for culture is limiting in clinical situations. Blood testing using the badger Tb ELISA test or the MAPIA 'Brock rapid test' (**194b**) has good specificity (94.3% and 95%, respectively), but poor sensitivity (40.7% and 53%, respectively). A badger gamma interferon test has improved sensitivity and specificity, but is not yet commercially available. The accepted 'gold standard' for Tb diagnosis in badgers is post-mortem examination and serial lymph node culture.

195 i. Tiletamine and zolazepam; ketamine and xylazine; ketamine and medetomidine; etorphine and acepromazine.

ii. Intramuscularly via a projectile syringe (to prevent a prolonged chase).

iii. Capture myopathy.

196 i. What are the likely causes of the injury in this hedgehog (196a)?
ii. How would you anaesthetize this animal in order to treat the wound?

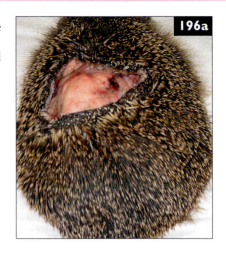

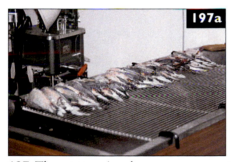

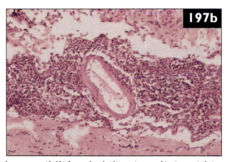

197 These mourning doves were presented to a wildlife rehabilitation clinic within a 48 hour period (197a). All 19 doves were thin to emaciated and all exhibited varying degrees of central nervous system signs on presentation, ranging from a mild ataxia to profound torticollis with rolling seizures. All received supportive nutritional care, diazepam and systemic anti-inflammatories, but died within 24 hours of presentation.

Gross necropsies revealed emaciation with little muscle mass and no fat stores. The kaolin linings of the ventriculi were all bright green, but no ingesta was present in the upper gastrointestinal (GI) tracts. No parasites were found in intestinal content or in scrapings of the GI mucosa. All other organs appear normal. Histopathology of the brain was performed on several of the birds (197b).

i. What is the significance of the histopathological lesion?
ii. How did these doves acquire this infection?
iii. Is this condition treatable?

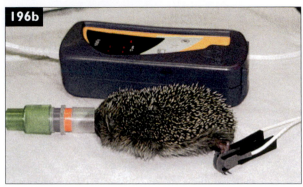

196 i. The linear wound is likely to have been caused by garden equipment, in particular a garden strimmer.

ii. General anaesthesia using a gaseous anaesthetic chamber. Isoflurane or sevoflurane are the gaseous agents of choice, the latter having the benefit of being less irritant to the mucous membranes. Once anaesthesia is induced, a close-fitting mask is placed over the nose and mouth to maintain anaesthesia. Small face masks are available, but alternatives can be adapted from existing anaesthetic equipment (196b). For longer procedures, hedgehogs should be intubated using a small laryngoscope to visualize the larynx before placing an uncuffed endotracheal tube (typically size 2.0 or 2.5).

Monitoring equipment can be used in small mammals (such as the pulse oximeter in 196b) and some commercial ventilators will work safely in animals of very low body weight. Temperature should be monitored and maintained.

197 i. There is a cross section of a nematode larva in the brain. Additional sections confirmed the identification of *Baylisascaris procyonis* larvae.

ii. By ingesting seeds found in raccoon faeces. Omnivorous raccoons eat mulberries and other fruits, the seeds of which pass through the GI tract undigested. Mourning doves and other ground-feeding seed-eaters subsequently ingest the seeds, which are contaminated with the first-stage larvated ova of *B. procyonis*, the raccoon roundworm.

iii. In an aberrant host, such as mourning doves, the *B. procyonis* larvae migrate out of the GI tract with an affinity for the brain and eye. The roundworms can be eliminated from the raccoon with most common anthelmintics (e.g. pyrantel pamoate or fenbendazole), but once an aberrant host has shown clinical signs, the damage done by the migrating larvae is irreversible.

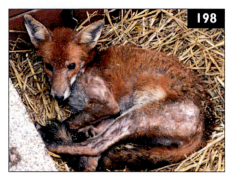

198 i. What condition is this red fox suffering from (198)?
ii. How would you confirm your diagnosis?
iii. What are your options for treating this condition in the fox, and what might influence your choice of treatment?

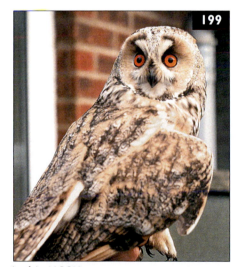

199 i. What species is this (199)?
ii. What considerations are important when considering post-treatment release of this species in the UK?

198 i. Chronic mange, caused by the parasite *Sarcoptes scabiei*. The animal shows generalized skin lesions, weight loss and debilitation. Mange is relatively common in foxes and appears to be especially prevalent in the urban fox population.

ii. By demonstration of *S. scabiei* mites on microscopic examination of deep skin scrapes taken when the fox is sedated or anaesthetized.

iii. This type of mange affects other canids, including domestic dogs. Several dog-licensed commercial spot-on preparations containing the active ingredients selamectin, moxidectin or amitraz are available for the treatment of mange in foxes. Other products, such as injected or oral ivermectin and topical amitraz baths, have also been used successfully in foxes. All these products have the disadvantage of requiring multiple (two plus) treatments for them to be fully effective, requiring the fox to remain in captivity or be re-trapped. Foxes with mange are often severely debilitated when presented for treatment, with possible underlying systemic disease. Euthanasia is the preferred course of action in the majority of cases. The effect of the treatment of individual chronic cases on the prevalence of the disease in the fox population as a whole is unknown.

199 i. A short-eared owl.

ii. The status of this species varies according to region. It is partially migratory, moving south in the winter from the northern parts of its range. For example, in the UK it is found all year round as a breeding species in the Midlands and further north. In the south it has tended to be a winter non-breeding migrant. However, this may be changing and can even vary from year to year. It is becoming clear in southern England that whereas most short-eared owls are seen in spring and autumn, there are more recent instances of this species being observed during the summer. Therefore, it is important that before releasing a short-eared owl its migratory status must be considered. If not fit to migrate, it should be retained in captivity until the next resident season. It is also important to liaise with local ornithologists to obtain information on the local status and movements of the species that year.

200 Fishing hook and/or line injuries are commonly seen in wild avian casualties and are particularly common in waterfowl. Ducks and swans may be seen with fishing line hanging from their bills. Bats may also fall victim to discarded or abandoned fishing tackle and are more likely to be found hanging from a branch after becoming snagged on fishing line. What advice should be given to members of the public who report such incidents?

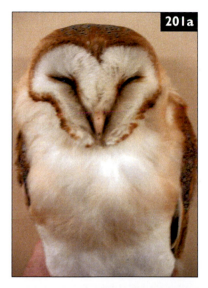

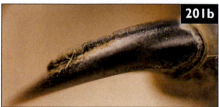

201 i. What species is this (201a, b)?
ii. What age and sex is this bird, and how can this be determined?

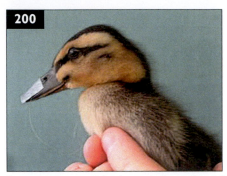

200 Care must be taken not to provide the member of public with advice that is likely to compromise their own safety. Great care is required when catching waterfowl on water and when handling large, potentially aggressive birds, such as swans, or when climbing trees and handling bats.

Where a bird is seen swallowing a fishing line, it should be caught in order to remove the fishing line and assess and treat any associated health problems. Members of the public should not attempt to do this and specialist wildlife rescue agencies should be contacted. Once captured, the line should be secured to the bird's bill to prevent further ingestion (**200**). Where a bat has been found snagged on discarded fishing tackle, it should be supported in a net while the fishing line is cut, if safe to do so. All bats are potential vectors of bat lyssavirus and should be handled as little as possible and with gloves. Scooping the bat into a small box or container minimizes the need for handling.

201 i. A barn owl.
ii. The lack of speckling on the breast feathers and the 'heart-shaped' facial disc indicate this is probably a male. Females tend to have much rounder facial discs and black speckling over the white breast feathers. **201b** shows the talon on the third digit. On this talon is a flange, indentations of which give an idea of the age. In this case the indentations are quite deep, showing this to be a bird older than two years. The width of the flange may also assist in sexing, although these differences are very subtle.

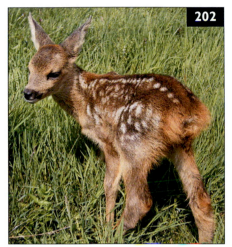

202 You are presented with a healthy roe deer kid (fawn) (202). How would you deal with this animal?

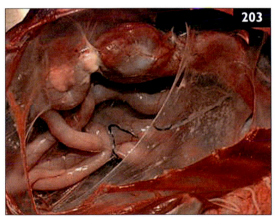

203 Air sac disease is not uncommonly identified at post-mortem examination in wild birds. What can be seen in the air sacs of this bird (203), and what is their significance?

202 Deer fawns are mistakenly found as 'orphans' when they have simply been left in cover and the doe is still nearby. It is unlikely that the fawn could be successfully returned to where found and accepted by its mother at this stage, but this should not be completely ruled out.

Deer fawns are difficult to rear, hard to release and may easily become imprinted during rearing. The prognosis for fawns brought into captivity is poor. Suitable facilities with experienced staff are required for rearing. Male hand-reared animals in particular can be aggressive and dangerous when adult. Hydration status should be assessed and fluid therapy administered as necessary. Bottle or syringe feeding is the ideal, but may be resented and stressful initially. Fawns may be persuaded to lap from a bucket or bowl. Milk should be fed every 3–4 hours until the fawn is 8–10 weeks old. Ewe or goat milk is best, with vitamin and probiotic supplementation. Defecation and urination should be stimulated by using warm damp cotton wool around the perineum. Fawns should be weaned at about ten weeks old. Suitable weaning foods include leafy browse (e.g. hawthorn, bramble, wild rose) and fruits, although commercial lamb food may also be fed. Hay and water should be provided.

203 Pentastomids, also known as tongue worms, a taxon of about 130 species of parasites living exclusively in the respiratory tracts of vertebrates. Pentastomids are vermiform, obligate parasites that are largely devoid of morphological features. They are generally white in colour, although the black intestine can be seen through the cuticle, and possess a mouth flanked by two paired hooks. Approximately 90% of pentastomid species infect the lungs of reptiles. Only two species have been identified as parasites of birds (*Reighardia sternae* in gulls and terns, and *Reighardia lomviae* [pictured here] in guillemots). Both species live in the host's air sacs and have a direct life cycle. A third avian pentastomid species was identified in the air sacs of a black vulture (*Aegypius monachus*). While the presence of pentastomid parasites in the air sacs may cause a low-grade irritation and airsacculitis, they are not regarded as a primary cause of death in marine birds. Secondary bacterial infections may worsen the clinical and pathological picture and this may become significant where birds are debilitated for other reasons such as oiling.

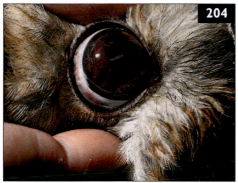

204 The eye of a tawny owl is shown (**204**).
i. What can be seen?
ii. What are this bird's prospects for release?

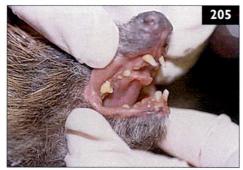

205 Dental disease is a common problem in captive hedgehogs (**205**), but it also affects those in the wild. Dental problems have been shown to be a significant cause of debilitation and death in hedgehogs that have been rehabilitated and released.
i. What factors might predispose to dental disease in this species?
ii. How might dental disease be prevented and treated in hedgehogs?

204 i. The anterior chamber is full of blood (hyphaema), probably as a result of trauma.

ii. It is unlikely that this bird will regain much, if any, vision in this eye. While tawny owls do use their sense of hearing for hunting, their sight, in particular binocular vision, is extremely important. This requires full vision in both eyes. Therefore, this bird has little prospect for release and euthanasia should be advised as soon as possible unless the bird can be kept in captivity in such accommodation that its welfare is not compromised.

205 i. The natural diet of hedgehogs is predominantly earthworms, molluscs and insects. The chitinous exoskeletons of insects probably protect the teeth to some extent against the build up of tartar and development of periodontal disease. 'Unnatural diets', such as those fed in captivity or found when hedgehogs are in proximity to humans, might be expected to predispose to the development of dental disease.

ii. The build up of tartar around and between the teeth leads to gingivitis, bacterial infection, gum regression, periodontal disease and, eventually, tooth loss. Treatment involves standard small animal dentistry techniques under general anaesthesia. Antibacterials, such as metronidazole (10–20 mg/kg q12h), should be used for 5–7 days, ideally starting courses of such drugs 24–48 hours before dental surgery. In captive hedgehogs the diet should be adapted to try and prevent recurrence of dental problems. Commercial insectivorous diets containing chitin are available. Hard foods, such as crushed cat biscuits, may be fed as a readily available alternative. Seaweed-based products added to food ('Plaque off®') and chlorhexidine solutions added to water may help to prevent periodontal disease. Where possible, advice should be given to members of the public feeding hedgehogs in their gardens as to the most appropriate feeds to use.

206 A male adult koala is presented to a wildlife clinic. The animal was found on the ground at the edge of a reserve with increased respiratory effort and ataxia. There was little resistance to restraint. On physical examination the koala was found to be in good body condition, weighing 5.7 kg. No abnormalities were detected on thoracic auscultation (206) or abdominal palpation. The left superficial axillary lymph node and both rostral mandibular lymph nodes were enlarged. However, the koala

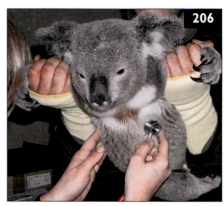

resented abdominal palpation. A blood sample was collected from the cephalic vein and haematology/biochemistry revealed the following results:

Parameter	Result	Reference range
Haemoglobin	70 g/l (7 g/dl)	88–140 (8.8–14.0)
PCV	0.21 l/l (21%)	0.29–0.44 (29–44)
MCHC	301 g/l (30.1 g/dl)	298–330 (29.8–33.0)
MCV	108 fl (108 mm³)	94–117 (94–117)
RBCs	1.6×10^{12}/l (1.6×10^6/μl)	2.7–4.2 (2.7–4.2)
WBCs	74×10^9/l (74×10^3/μl)	2.8–11.2 (2.8–11.2)
Neutrophils	12.5×10^9/l (12.5×10^3/μl)	0.5–6.3 (0.5–6.3)
Lymphocytes	61×10^9/l (61×10^3/μl)	0.2–5.8 (0.2–5.8)
Monocytes	0.5×10^9/l (0.5×10^3/μl)	0.0–0.6 (0.0–0.6)
Eosinophils	0×10^9/l (0×10^3/μl)	0.0–1.1 (0.0–1.1)
Urea	7.1 mmol/l (19.9 mg/dl)	0.2–6.6 (0.56–18.48)
Creatinine	0.11 mmol/l (0.0012 mg/dl)	0.08–0.15 (0.0009–0.0017)
AST	151 u/l	0–134
ALT	144 u/l	(0–236)
ALP	38 u/l	(25–219)
GGT	25 u/l	(0–16)
LDH	401 u/l	(79–412)
Total protein	60 g/l (6.0 g/dl)	58–83 (5.8–8.3)
Albumin	29 g/l (2.9 g/dl)	34–50 3.4–5.0)
Globulins	31 g/l (3.1 g/dl)	18–39 (1.8–3.9)
Calcium	2.76 mmol/l (11.04 mg/dl)	2.28–2.97 (9.12–11.88)
I. phosphate	1.23 mmol/l (3.81 mg/dl)	0.79–1.96 (2.45–6.08)

i. What is the likely diagnosis?
ii. How would you confirm the diagnosis?
iii. What treatment options are available?
iv. Which virus is this disease associated with?

206 i. Lymphoid neoplasia. The marked lymphocytosis is highly suggestive of this common disease of koalas. Supporting clinical features include peripheral lymphadenopathy, moderate anaemia and mild hypoalbuminaemia.

ii. Excisional biopsy of one of the enlarged superficial lymph nodes may reveal neoplastic lymphocytes. Alternatively, a bone marrow aspirate can be collected from the ileal crest under general anaesthesia. Squash preparations of the aspirate are evaluated microscopically for myeloid:erythroid ratio, which in a healthy koala should be 1.7 (0.8–2.7). If the koala is euthanased or dies, a post-mortem examination will permit definitive diagnosis via histopathology of multiple organs.

iii. No successful treatment options have been reported. Chemotherapy has been attempted in selected cases, but as yet the results have been disappointing.

iv. Koala retrovirus (KoRV), an endogenous retrovirus closely related to gibbon ape leukaemia virus, is associated with a number of common diseases of the koala, including lymphoid neoplasia. Koalas with confirmed lymphoid neoplasia frequently have high circulating levels of KoRV RNA.

Appendix: Common and Latin names

African buffalo	*Syncerus caffer*
American alligator	*Alligator mississippiensis*
American crow	*Corvus brachyrhynchos*
American mink	*Neovison vison*
Arabian oryx	*Oryx leucoryx*
Arctic fox	*Alopex lagopus*
Atlantic white-sided dolphin	*Lagenorhynchus acutus*
Badger (European)	*Meles meles*
Bald eagle	*Haliaceetus leucocephalus*
Barn owl	*Tyto alba*
Bat-eared fox	*Otocyon megalotis*
Bennett's wallaby	*Macropus rufogriseus rufogriseus*
Bewick's swan	*Cygnus columbianus*
Bison	*Bison bison*
Blackbird	*Turdus merula*
Black-headed gull	*Larus ribundus*
Blacksmith plover	*Anitibyx armatus*
Black vulture	*Aegypius monachus*
Blue hare	*Lepus timidus*
Blue jay	*Cyanocitta cristata*
Bonelli's eagle	*Hieraaetus fasciatus*
Brown hare	*Lepus europaeus*
Brush-tailed possum	*Trichosurus vulpecula*
Canada goose	*Branta canadensis*
Chaffinch	*Fringilla coelebs*
Chimpanzee	*Pan troglodytes*
Chuck-will's-widow	*Caprimulgus carolinensis*
Collared dove	*Streptopelia decaocto*
Common blackbird	*Turdus merula*
Common buzzard	*Buteo buteo*
Common cuckoo	*Cuculus canorus*
Common dolphin	*Delphinus delphis*
Common goldeneye	*Bucephala clangula*
Common kestrel	*Falco tinnunculus*
Coot	*Fulica* spp.
Cottontail rabbit	*Silvilagus floridanus*
Daubenton's bat	*Myotis daubentonii*

Desert tortoise	*Gopherus agassizii*
Eastern bearded dragon	*Pogona barbata*
Eastern box turtle	*Terrapene carolina carolina*
Eastern chipmunk	*Tamias striatus*
Eastern grey squirrel	*Sciurus carolinensis*
Eastern pipistrelle	*Pipistrellus subflavus*
Elephant	*Loxodonta* spp.
Elk	*Cervus elaphus*
Flamingo	*Phoenicopterus* spp.
Florida manatee	*Trichecus manatus latirostris*
Fox	*Vulpes vulpes*
Fox squirrel	*Sciurus niger*
Golden pheasant	*Chrysolophus pictus*
Goldfinch	*Carduelis carduelis*
Grey squirrel	*Sciurus carolinensis*
Great blue heron	*Ardea herodias*
Great horned owl	*Bubo virginianus*
Great northern diver	*Gavia immer*
Great horned owl	*Bubo virginianus*
Greater flamingo	*Phoenicopterus roseus*
Greenfinch	*Carduelis chloris*
Green turtle	*Chelonia mydas*
Grey fox	*Urocyon cinereoargenteus*
Grey seal	*Halichoerus grypus*
Guillemot	*Uria aalge*
Harbour porpoise	*Phocoena phocoena*
Hare	*Lepus* spp.
Hedgehog (European)	*Erinaceus europaeus*
Hippopotamus	*Hippopotamus amphibius*
Houbara bustard	*Chlamydotis undulata*
House sparrow	*Passer domesticus*
Impala	*Aepyceros malampus*
Jackass penguin	*Spheniscus demersus*
Koala	*Phascolarctos cinereus*
Kori bustard	*Ardeotis kori*
Loggerhead sea turtle	*Caretta caretta*

Long-finned pilot whale	*Globicephala melas*
Long-tailed duck	*Clangula hyemalis*
Mallard	*Anas platyrhynchos*
Moorhen	*Gallinula chloropus*
Mountain gorilla	*Gorilla berengei berengei*
Mourning dove	*Zenaida macroura*
Mute swan	*Cygnus olor*
Osprey	*Pandion haliaetus*
Otter (Eurasian)	*Lutra lutra*
Pacific harbour seal	*Phoca vitulina richardsi*
Pallas cat	*Felis manul*
Peregrine falcon	*Falco peregrinus*
Pipistrelle bat	*Pipistrellus pipistrellus*
Prairie falcon	*Falco mexicanus*
Rabbit	*Oryctolagus cuniculi*
Raccoon	*Procyon lotor*
Raccoon dog	*Nyctereutes procyonoides*
Rainbow lorikeet	*Trichoglossus haematodus*
Red bat	*Lasiurus borealis*
Red fox	*Vulpes vulpes*
Red kangaroo	*Macropus rufus*
Red squirrel	*Sciurus vulgaris*
Red-tailed hawk	*Buteo jamaicensis*
Reindeer	*Rangifer tarandus*
Roe deer	*Capreolus capreolus*
Rosenberg's goanna	*Varanus rosenbergi*
Sage grouse	*Centrocercus urophasianus*
Saker falcon	*Falco cherrug*
Scaly-breasted lorikeet	*Trichoglossus chlorolepidotus*
Scimitar-horned oryx	*Oryx dammah*
Seal (Common/ Harbour)	*Phoca vitulina*
Serotine bat	*Eptesicus serotinus*
Shelduck	*Tadorna tadorna*
Short-beaked echidna	*Tachyglossus aculeatus*
Short-eared owl	*Asio flammeus*
Shrew (Common/ Eurasian)	*Sorex araneus*
Silver-haired bat	*Lasionycteris noctivagans*
South American forest rabbit	*Sylvilagus brasiliensis*
Sparrowhawk (Northern/Eurasian)	*Accipiter nisus*
Stock dove	*Columba oenas*
Stone curlew	*Burhinus oedicnemius*
Striped skunk	*Mephitis mephitis*
Tawny owl	*Strix aluco*
Vampire bat	*Desmodus rotundus*
Western grey kangaroo	*Dacelo novaeguineae*
Western grey squirrel	*Sciurus griseus*
White-backed vulture	*Gyps bengalensis*
White-bellied bustard	*Eupodotis senegalensis*
White-tailed deer	*Odocoileus virginianus*
Whooper swan	*Cygnus cygnus*
Woodchuck	*Marmota monax*
Yellow mongoose	*Cynictis penicillata*

Index

Index

Index

Index